I Flew

The Cuckoo's Nest

The Madhouse Memoirs

DR CHRISTOPHER FORD

Fisher King Publishing

I Flew Into The Cuckoo's Nest

Published by
Fisher King Publishing
www.fisherkingpublishing.co.uk

An element of the cover image is courtesy of franckreporter

This book is dedicated to my family, Susan, Jessica, and Jojo, who have (somehow) managed to put up with the constant sight of me hunched over a laptop trying to write books for the last year. Thank you xxx

I also thank Rick and all at Fisher King for publishing my books, you are very brave!

Contents

Preamble

I can only pray you didn't buy this book in the hope it will inspire. It won't. Not if you are thinking of becoming a carer, a nurse, or any kind of social services employee helping the mentally ill or those with learning disabilities. It really won't inspire you. I am sure there are plenty of other books that will, and I am equally sure there are many reasons to be inspired for such valuable and rewarding work. Please don't let me put you off, I hope you kept the receipt.

This is a 'warts an' all' account of a career lasting around twelve years at the sharp end of such services, mainly under lock and key. Warts 'an all, meaning the Warts, plus the Halitosis and the Skid-Marks. I am not sugar coating anything nor purposefully embellishing. Words, in dialogue, have been used to the best of my ability to replicate what I remember but they may well differ to the original experience. It starts in the 1980's and, looking back, it may as well have been in the Victorian age, such was the madness, misery, and mayhem.

Obviously, I have been damaged, these years (mis) shaped me. I've become cynical, developed a few ticks and neuroses; it drives you mad eventually. I have been left somewhat cold and fairly devoid of particular emotions or empathy - or so I'm sometimes informed. I don't have much time for people wallowing in self-pity. Having said that, I am now left with a proneness to social anxiety, which is probably part of my own deep mind wallowing in self-pity, go figure.

I can't fluff it up into something it wasn't. You can't put lipstick on a pig and get away with it, it's still obviously a pig, so why bother? It was mainly hell, interspersed with lots of drink and drug fuelled nights to numb the mind and force some cathartic laughter.

Every event in this book happened. You may think otherwise, but I assure they did. Names, locations, and stories have been mixed up or swapped with others to avoid upsetting anyone who may think they are mis-characterised, you haven't been, and it's not you!

There have been many occasions when I have heard people talk about certain experiences they've had regarding people with mental health issues, or the institutions they may have inhabited. I've nearly always thought, 'Jeez, is that it?' I'm not so competitive as to believe my stories are better, or more mind-blowing, but they usually are!

I know that if I start with one event, I will have to go on to recall another, and they always have too much of a back story so I get that I can't be bothered, I don't go there. I literally say, 'Oh! Don't get me started!' like an old housewife comparing husbands with her neighbour over the garden fence. Either that or I don't want to get into that game of bettering your opponent's anecdotes.

You end up not listening to each other as you wait to get your next one in.

I've not actually told anyone most of these stories, not even my wife until she offered to go through it, while shouting, 'No Way! You're making this up, surely.'

For some reason, I've always not been motivated enough to start the tale. It's a bit like having a burning and brilliant question in a science class but knowing the complexity of such a question would require a drawn-out monologue, you shy away from putting your hand up. Or having the best 'Englishman, Irishman and Scotsman walk into a pub' joke ever, an ideal opportunity for you to jump in and make everyone laugh, boosting your ego, but you just can't bring yourself to start it. Too long, too much attention, likely to balls it up - do it another time. But you don't. So, I listen to such memoirs of others and if they ask me for mine, I more often change the subject.

Obviously, there are many others with careers in this field who have similar experiences, and through the same period I recount here, some are still doing their jobs. Hats off to them for persevering, surviving even. Where would our disadvantaged be if it wasn't for those who step up to care; they deserve far more than they get paid.

But if you are not planning to enter this world, keen as mustard, all wet behind the ears, and full of fluffy dreams, then read on.

Welcome To The Cuckoo's Nest

Nothing quite prepares you for some of the characters in Psychiatric hospitals, even more so in forensic units. Offenders. These are specialist centres where you try to filter the mad from the bad. Do they require treatment or punishment? Are they mentally ill or mentally impaired, or a bit of both? Are they of sound enough mind to be responsible for their behaviour? Are they pretending not to be? Acute admissions and assessment, half secure lock-up seclusion, half open (with strict rules).

One such unit was where I first worked as a Registered Staff Nurse. This meant I was expected to be in charge in the absence of the Charge Nurse, who was often absent. As were a lot of staff, regularly.

We were very well trained in 'Control and Restraint' (C&R), including the fully-tooled-up riot helmet, shield, and body armour techniques, I will reveal some later. Interestingly, one violent person required three C&R trained staff; two seriously fighting required six minimum, we never had six, and often not the three. An alarm could sound for reinforcements from other units within the massive grounds but whatever mayhem ensued usually fizzled out by the time they came – fighting is pretty tiring. Having said that, psychosis seems to have that Incredible Hulk effect.

We had them all in – the mad, the bad, the impaired,

the ill, and all the ones in that massive grey area. The inmates from prison, the accused from police cells, and the patients from hospitals, sectioned (section 36 of the mental health act), or not – we had 'em all in stock. Most were somewhat messed up on drugs, prescribed or not, either way they could be psychotic and violent, or zombified catatonics, sex offenders, murderers, or just your friendly stabbers, and arsonists. Robbers and thieves made up the semi-secure gang who had gained enough trust to work on the hospital farm – until they got cross and smashed up the hospital farm shop (a care in the community initiative) with mattocks. You could set your watch to some.

I won't tell you what he was in for just yet, but Jeff James was a one-off. The initiator and centre stage of most jaw-droppingly serious incidents. Not his real name of course, but it was a similar alliteration, in fact I can think right now of four people with poetic alliteration names who will feature in this book – it must be a thing in that part of the world, maybe a dodgy gene passing around for parents who need it as a prompt?

Anyway, Jeff. A thick Geordie accent from the back streets of Newcastle. Thick, as in 'Thick.' The deportment of a male silverback – probably a little less intelligent. Head on, rear facing, and profile views were all 'Gorilla,' a more 'Gorillic' human you would be pushed to beat.

Palms pointing backwards, revealed fingers dark black

hairy to the extremities, for some reason always curled in a semi fist. The hyper-lordotic lumber spine went from a fully vertical back to a near horizontal upper arse, you could have put a small saddle on him. Imagine the half-man, half-goat 'faun,' in Greek mythology – actually, scrub that, imagine a Gorilla. To call him 'thick set' is an understatement and a little disparaging to yoghurt. His wildly placed facial hair was like wire, jet black, and it used to bounce as he walked. His one eyebrow resembled a nasty poisonous caterpillar from Borneo. The five o'clock shadow bloomed at midday sharp. Back of the head hair stopped around the Achilles tendons as he didn't shave what he couldn't see. He also had a bum chin complete with a deep dimple, a minute but dark and hairy scary place (things would surely live in there). Thick Set, pure muscle, rock hard. Unusually, he liked to wear a suit, it always looked tight. He would always start fights and sometimes scrap so hard, others would need weapons, his suit would become ripped extensively, and blood splattered. He wore said suit with pride, the rips and blood were medals – they communicated 'you should see the state of the other guy.' He would wear the rags for weeks until someone gave him a replacement – never his fault of course. A new suit would calm him for a while.

Always started fights and arguments, always found something calm and peaceful to stir up. This was pre-woke sensitivity, anything and everything triggered him.

DR CHRISTOPHER FORD

A compliment would offend.

"Good morning, Jeff."

"What the fuck's that supposed to mean?" Here we go.

A classic Jeffery James incident... It was 7am when I ran into the office for hand-over from the night shift, I was groggy from the late, beery, night before and, to be fair, a tad fragile. Barely awake, I was surprised and pleased to see two young female student nurses politely and nervously waiting for me. Suddenly I felt alive. They sat through 'hand-over' looking very concerned when hearing about potential incidents with some of our ticking time bombs. We gave them reassurance and a tour of the seclusion cells via the battered steel door.

Others went to stir the inmates as I sat with them over coffee to brief and inform. Basic dos and don'ts. The key message was – IF THERE IS ANY VIOLENCE, BE CALM AND JUST LET US DEAL WITH IT, WE ARE VERY WELL TRAINED AND EQUIPPED, IT MAY BE A LITTLE SHOCKING BUT WE ARE IN TOTAL CONTROL.

Breakfast went without incident, most inmates/patients (I gather they are called 'service users' now) were up and fed, most were also fed up (did you see what I did there?), the TV was on, and everyone was well into their fourth fag. I was just about to do the drug round. Maybe a chance to impress the students with my pharmaceuticals.

The first inkling was muffled shouting from the dorms

upstairs, the male one. Then a massive crash, a wardrobe ripped from its security screws, smashing on the heavily worn and stained flooring that was once a nice calming patterned carpet. Then a scream and echoic verbal abuse coming down the stairwell, ever louder, and travelling my way. OK, one of these mornings, I thought, way too early for a fight.

Expecting Jeff to make a whirlwind appearance, I was rather surprised to see the ginger haired and heavily tattooed (rare in those days) Adam Abbott – yup another double letter. Adam had his moments, very aggressive, very violent, but fair with it. You could usually tell when he was stirring and often de-escalate with a bit of a chat.

If Adam had long periods of non-aggression, he would play football with me in our hospital team (home games only). Local Sunday league – we quite often went down to ten, and then to nine if I had to drag him back to the unit. Often agreeing that his kicking the ref was justified.

Back to the chaos.

Adam charged right at me, very quickly. No chance of 'decking him' as I was stuck between another staff member and a sofa with wooden armrests. I got forearmed in the face and fell back onto the sofa with my head hitting the wall and an armrest digging into my right scapula.

I was wearing a shirt, as was the rules, and Adam managed to grab the front of the collar in a twist while falling on top of me. Another 'patient' (let's go with that term from now on) started screaming and that triggered another to throw coffee mugs at the wall. My colleague went to deal with that. In this situation I would normally be able to get a hold or a pinch somewhere strategic, that would allow an escape. I was manoeuvring my left hand into position while using my right to take pressure away from my throat, breathing was difficult. Adam had mad wild eyes; he was spraying spit in my face while shouting God knows what - something had really set him off.

Jeff.

A matter of seconds later; cue Jeff. "You bastard, fucking bastard, cunt," he bellowed, all Geordie like, as he leapt through the air, and landed on the back of Adam. He seemed to be trying to help me but was too stupid to realise his ample weight had added to the force that completely shut off my airways and foiled any bid for escape. Two big heavy bodies on top of me, I felt the sofa collapse and the armrest snap.

At this moment I started to lose consciousness.

Spoiler alert! People say as you drift off to death, your life flashes through your mind, you see loved ones, you think of how you wish you could say goodbye, maybe admit to the odd misdemeanour, seek forgiveness... No, that's not what happens.

You think, 'How fucking embarrassing,' I could see the two nurses watching in horror. Just two minutes ago I was flirting with them, impressing them, and now I'm dying right in front of them, pathetically.

I tried to make eyes that said, OK you can definitely react now! Like call for help, raise the alarm, hit these two fuckers on the head with a chair, anything!

I could see them frozen, expecting me to regain control as explained, but no, a greyness appeared. My vision was going and then it did. I was still thinking, 'how embarrassing,' as I died.

As a child, I saw a picture of Dr Bently's leg, surrounded by charred carpet and a walking aid. Spontaneous Human Combustion. I was afraid that I would, one day, spontaneously combust. Not worried at all about dying from it, but incredibly worried about how embarrassing that would be.

Obviously, I didn't die. Apparently, the sofa collapsed some more, and we all fell to the floor. Adam let go of my body, Jeff started hitting him with the broken arm rest, and he bolted through a French window, across the football pitch, and on the run. AWOL.

I came round, the police were called, and I was taken to hospital. No lasting damage, lots of bruising, a couple weeks off and eventually a couple thousand pounds compensation. Hoorah.

Several weeks later I was asked to provide photographic evidence of bruising. Old bruising. I found greens, yellows and a purple eyeshadow worked best.

Jeff James. He appears quite a lot in this book. Oh, and

I forgot to say what he was in for.

Work.

He was a nurse.

Testing The Water

It was one of those jobs, or careers that I fell into. We lived near three old institutions, 'Loony-bins.' For some reason the powers that controlled psychiatry decided our town needed to be sandwiched between two sprawling and rather scary looking camps for the mentally challenged. I remember with my friends driving past or on the bus, nearly everyone childish enough would pull all kinds of contortions and make noises, making fun of whatever poor souls resided within the walls.

This was the mid-eighties. Not that long ago, not quite Bedlam, but not far off. Notions of decency and compassion had led to significant human rights and changes in how the community should welcome back into society, people with, let's say, 'disorders.' Having said that, the local people still used the terms spastics, divvies, and mongs, while the professional establishment used 'backward,' 'cripple,' 'invalid,' and 'retarded.' When later qualified and working in a specialist unit, I once read a referral letter from one consultant to our service asking if we could assess the 'leprechaun in his care.' I could only but laugh.

They were still largely excluded from society, living in large cold buildings, shared dorms and, in rare cases, but something I witnessed, a communal hose down, lined up naked and 'high-pressure' shot at, before breakfast.

'They enjoyed it,' I was persuaded. It was clear that some older inmates had originally been incarcerated for anti-social behaviours such as pregnancy out of wedlock. This immorality must have been due to a mental defect, they declared, (allowed under The Mental Deficiency Act, 1913), so initially without a real mental disorder, but ultimately an inherited one - called institutionalisation. Legend had it that one such incarceration, without the pregnancy element, I think, was a close relative of Queen Elizabeth II, not that I ever saw any evidence.

I knew a couple of friends who worked in these 'bins,' they were either catering or maintenance staff and they all had stories. One described a monster of a woman who was in the 'hospital unit.'

We were in a noisy pub, he excitedly shouted, "Guess what she's in for."

"What?" we shouted back.

"Fucking bestiality man!" he declared, before 'verifying' she definitely shagged horses – turns out he misheard the clinical staff over breakfast, and it was 'obesity.' To be fair, he was a bit of a simpleton himself, it was a rural area, lots of thumbs on elbows, a place where your mother could also be your aunty. Maybe that's why local facilities were abundant.

The Stiff

I remember being told the story of the night transfer to the mortuary (yes, these bins had their own mortuaries).

It was a cold winter's night, (are you sitting comfortably?) the entire hospital was deep in snow, a blizzard in full swing, you couldn't distinguish the gravel roads between residential blocks from the grassy lawned areas and the steep banks falling into darkness. An inmate had died suddenly in one isolated block situated at the top of a hill. Two burley men on their night shift were called to transport the body down to the mortuary, vehicles were out of the question so they decided a hospital trolley bed would be the best bet, they could half carry, half drag it through the drifts, no problem. They managed to get the body onto the bed with some dignity, supine with a blanket on top. No doubt fellow inmates were watching in horror.

Everything was going smoothly, they managed to feel the path underfoot, and ploughed through, getting into a good stride and rhythm. Things started to go awry when gravity became involved. Always factor in gravity... and ice!

They turned a corner at some speed, one desperately trying to hold the weight while the other trying to steer with one hand while operating a torch with the other, they had hit sheer ice and were plummeting downhill like three Eddie the Eagles, but not pointing in the direction in which they were traveling. The torch was knocked out of hand as they hit a kerb hard. The burley chaps smacked into each other and into the cold hard steel of the trolley, everything came to a hard and immediate stop. Except the body.

Apparently, even after finding the torch, they couldn't locate it. The steep slope descended into a darkness of heavy snow. The blizzard increased, they were battered and bruised, it was well into the early hours; mission aborted, for now.

No worries, in the morning, in the light, and hopefully in better weather they will complete their task.

It was a lovely start to the day, blue skies, white pristine grounds, and convenient tracks had been created some hours before leading back up to the site of the accident.

They got to the obvious markings of a crash location, looked down the steep bank and there it was, the body, wrapped around a tree.

Moderate rigor mortis sets in in a few hours; meat freezes around the same time, attempting to place a stiff body supine or prone when it is stuck in the kind of position you see a child learning to dive at the poolside, is futile. They looked like the deliverers of statues when entering the mortuary.

It had to fit into a cold storage unit, like the ones you see on TV with labelled toes sticking out.

Apparently, they needed heavy tools, and burly men prepared to do something they never, in their wildest macabre dreams, imagined.

The anti-climax to this story came about four years later, and again another two years later, when I was told the same story in different establishments in other areas of the country. In fact, I finished the story off for them on the latter occasion. Whether mine was the original, true, passed around and claimed by others, tale, or it was an old industry fable, I've no idea.

Why Though? Are You Mad?

I was in need of some income and direction having returned from a very eventful frolic around the Middle East as a nineteen-year-old. I hadn't become the rock star as expected, the band was still going but more sideways than any other positive direction. I also needed to fund my rent and social life, while knowing that I could fall into a life of drug taking and nothingness without structure. I messed up my A levels and thought a qualification of some sort worth gaining. I had another mate who worked as a nursing assistant before signing up to be a registered mental nurse, he was getting good money and was living a wild existence in the nurses' accommodation they provided – it was full of nurses, female ones, with nurse uniforms. It also sounded fairly interesting.

I chose the one with more letters. RNMH, not RMN. Bound to be more prestigious, with more money. A decision I came to regret when only learning what the difference was when I was actually on the course. That was what the course did, it educated you about the difference between Mental Handicap, as was the 'H' at the time, and Mental Illness. I thought it was all in one bag. Being young and naïve and so politically incorrect, I didn't want to be wiping arses and dealing with those who dribbled. I was more interested in those who thought they were Napoleon. Within weeks, I was wiping arses.

Literally, by 7:10 am I would find myself lifting a disfigured body that made awful noises out of a stinking soaked bed, wiping their arses, washing them down, and padding them up before wheeling them into the breakfast room. No health and safety, manual handling courses, or robotic hoists, just imagine a very large sack of potatoes. Obviously, that was the short straw. Before starting my course, I was offered an immediate start as a nursing assistant on the ward that had the most disabled of bodies – Block 2. They don't exist in some countries – despite being born. Obviously, some had a degree of a 'quality of life,' others, I doubt, despite our attempts to jolly them along. I remember one Christmas, a quadriplegic (by means of no limbs) resident with barely any sight, or hearing, in a near vegetative state, was given a lovely present from some charity that dumped bags of random stuff off. It was a Filofax.

Different; I guess you can only have so many hats.

The unit where I worked probably had twenty beds, they were all occupied by twenty very badly physically and mentally disabled beings, bar two, who were obviously compos mentis to a degree, but wheelchair-bound and unable to speak or perform any self-care. They had a relationship with each other, one would blink at the other and receive happy grunts back. We understood at least some of their needs.

The day would go like this; get your allocated patients

up, 'toileted,' washed and dressed. Wheel them into the breakfast room. Serve them food or fill up their nasal feed bags. Go for your own breakfast in the huge staff canteen. Smoke a fag. Have coffee. Wheel the patients into a different room where telly was on (daytime TV was like a bad dream back then, simply awful – I still become disturbed when thinking of Pebble Mill at One). If budget allowed, we could take them out for a wheel, sometimes going to town or the beach in the 'Happy Ladybirds' minibus. In my first week, I went out with a couple of other nursing assistants and three patients in their chairs, completely oblivious. We went to the beach where the hospital had access to a beach hut. On this occasion we were dropped off by the minibus as it was being used later that day. Still very young and wet behind the ears, I thought it was completely ok for us all to get totally pissed out of our heads. The other staff pulled their bottles of gin and tonic and fags out from their ample handbags as if it was the done thing. I remember when it was time to get to our rendezvous with the bus, one of the nursing assistants tried to push their occupied wheelchair over some sand, where they flipped over leaving the patient face down and her laughing her head off and wetting herself. Not the Tuesday afternoon I was expecting, but quite a laugh – didn't quite seem right though. Sure enough, on return Matron went ballistic at us, although, being the early eighties, nothing to be too concerned about. Try not to drink so much next time, Matron advised. Turned out Matron was jealous.

Back to the routine, another 'toileting session,' e.g., wiping arses and changing massive pads, lunch, more sitting about before tea, more toileting, and then plonking them back into their high-sided beds. We had maybe four on shift plus a cook and a janitor, we would squabble over which patients we would have to prepare, some were easier than others, some less smelly. As a male, I was always given the biggest ones, and they were usually the most difficult to clean and, therefore the most messy – I could only do that part of the work whilst holding my breath, so in short bursts. I hated it.

It was a stupidly long shift. Twelve and a half hours. 07:00 to 19:30, allowing thirty mins handover to the night shift, they did the opposite 19:00 to 07:30. When I was offered the job, after a very brief interview, I couldn't get my head around such a long shift and such an early start. In fact, my very first shift was the start of a lifelong insomnia problem. I had gone out the night before, had a few beers, came home around 10 pm to get a good night's sleep. I needed to be alert the next day, up at 06:00. I so freaked out about having to appear keen and able in my new job that I did not sleep one minute, 06:00 hurtled towards me and my anxiety grew with each passing hour. I was a total wreck the next day, looked shit, and felt shit. Before that night I was happy-go-lucky, slept like a baby and now almost forty years on, I still suffer with the same neurosis. Self-fulfilling prophecy, 'better get to sleep now or you will look and feel shit the next day,' as soon as that thought hits me, I'm done for.

On day one, whilst feeling awful, I got the new boy initiations. Fell for it twice. "Chris mate, we have a problem with our scales, they need a special weight, can you go up to block twelve and ask them for a 'long weight'? They will be expecting you." A ten-minute walk up the hill was quite a nice break. I was met at block twelve by some smoking staff, all part of the gang, smiling strangely.

"Come for the long weight 'ave ya? Wait there."

I waited, and waited until I realised, I was having the 'long wait.' Bastards. HA HA HA HA HA yes, really funny, I agreed on my return while looking like crap and desperate to sleep.

An hour later, the feeding bag contraption had collapsed, apparently. This was a fairly urgent issue, and I was sent up to the maintenance department to get a 'long stand.' Bastards.

I've never clock-watched so many times and had such a long, hard day as that one. Money was good though, so I persevered. I had five weeks of it before starting my training at the local city 'School of Nursing.'

Thin Vessel

I was offered an opportunity though; take some patients on a holiday for a week, get double pay, and a whole week off to compensate. Holiday; hmmm sounds ominous. 24/7 care. But then a whole week off – paid.

'Where?'

The Kennet and Avon Canal. From Bath eastward through the Somerset countryside towards Reading, on a canal barge. Sounded brilliant. It was late spring, getting warm, everything blooming, the perfect antidote to the smells and noises of Block 2. We were taking three patients (lads, they said) from other units, and I was going with two other blokes who I barely knew but they seemed a laugh.

There were many blocks within the hospital, some contained patients who were much more able, could communicate, had personalities, and gave something back. I was really looking forward to working with these beings in my posts during training and eventually managing. I hated my short straw. For now, I would holiday with some.

Bryce was a staff nurse from New Zealand, definitely one of the 'in crowd.' He famously had wild sex with another staff nurse, who liked to flaunt her massive breasts and suspendered thighs, in the nurses' accommodation, and left her tied up on a bed on all fours, whilst he went to the pub. She had to bellow loud enough, and long enough, like some chained bovine beast, to raise help from the janitor who had lucked out with a sight and memory to satisfy him until his dying day. Maybe it was more of a James Herriot experience, who knows.

Alan was a large, beardy, seafaring type. I imagine a Morris dancer, or shanty singer, when not at work running the 'entertainment and activities' department out of the sports hall / staff pub. The idea was that he would make the inmates' lives more entertaining and stimulating, but it just became a smoke-filled area with pool tables that served as a knocking shop for drunken staff. For some reason, the place operated as a staff pub all day, well before licensing hours allowed 'all day' service. I think it was something to do with it being a 'club' for those in the nocturnal world of the 'emergency services.' Alcohol was tolerated in the hospital, probably because the hospital manager, another with an alliteral name, let's call him Bill Bonnet (obviously long gone by now, as are most characters in the book, but I guess relatives still exist), was a raving alcoholic with a bright red face and permanent shakes, always off sick, and when not, he could rarely be found if needed.

Very kindly, they loaded up at the hospital and arranged to come and pick me up from my home, I was looking forward to meeting the 'lads' from the other blocks, for obvious reasons we weren't taking any females.

As soon as I got into the bus, there was a strong smell of whiskey – and urine. Immediate red flags.

The 'lads' turned out to be patients equally as disabled as the lot I worked with, completely chairbound and doubly incontinent. Fuck's sake. I can only guess there was a massively accrued activity budget.

After an initial, "Hey, how's it going?" and, "All ready?" I found my little fold down seat, next to the wheelchairs that were fixed into the fittings that connected the (now removed) seating.

"Wrreeaahh."

'What was that?'

"Wrreeaahh."

It happened again, twenty seconds later.

"Wrreeaahh."

A horrible whiney groan, coming from my left. One of the 'lads,' emitting the most unpleasant noise you could wish for. So awful, it took me twenty minutes and several attempts to actually spell it.

"Is he ok?" I asked, thinking he may have got a finger stuck in the wheel clamps.

"Ah, that's David, don't worry about it mate, you will get used to it soon and barely notice. Wanna swig?" said Bryce. He wasn't the driver. Turned out, I wished he was.

"Wrreeaahh."

"Wrreeaahh."

"Wrreeaahh."

"AAAAAAAAAGGHH!"

"What the fuck was that?"

"That's Andy, sorry mate, he does that every now and again."

"Wrreeaahh." (Every twenty seconds – like a low battery beep in your fire alarms, you know it's coming but it always makes you jump)

The whiskey was lovely.

Alan was in a terrible mood; I think his wife just found out he was shagging someone else. You would have thought she'd be too busy washing up and darning socks to concern herself with his private life.

His driving was hell, everything done with aggression, I had to ask him to stop to be sick. "Lightweight," Bryce said, waving the second bottle of single malt at me. Both had fags on the go.

I would lean in towards their smoke to ease the smell of piss.

"Wrreeaahh, Wrreeaahh, Wrreeaahh."

"AAAAAAAAAGGHH!"

"Wrreeaahh."

When we arrived at the pick-up point it started to rain, it didn't stop raining the whole time we were afloat.

"You cook, I'll drive," said Alan.

"Fuck that," said Bryce, "you will just crash us on day one."

"Mate, who's more senior? Get those steaks going,"

Alan barked.

They bickered like a miserable man and wife. The boat was confined, cluttered, cold, and humid and it was pissing down outside. Oh joy.

"Wrreeaahh."

Alan and I, in large, yellow sou'westers, got the engine started, worked out the various levers and controls, and set off, sharing a joint. I felt happy. It didn't last.

The 'lads,' due to the weather were confined indoors.

"Wrreeaahh."

We had very little room to manoeuvre their bodies to change and wash them, the whole boat stank to high heaven by the evening. There were bags of soiled pads everywhere, we couldn't dump them until we got to the next stop off point, which was often hours.

Our first stop was next to a pub, where we decided to rotate shifts for the poor soul staying on ship.

Bryce didn't get the steaks on due to the sulk he was in, so we had a welcome pub meal, with takeaways for the 'boys.' Then we got the beers in.

I say first stop; it was our only stop.

That night we sat in the galley drinking whiskey, smoking joints, and listening to the music they brought. It was really good. I was a punk at the time, loved dub reggae and was yet to delve into some of the prepunk stuff from the seventies; other than Slade and Sweet, who I first got into before the Sex Pistols and The Clash etc.

We listened to Zuma by Neil Young and Crazy Horse, and also Moondance by Van Morrison – I really loved those albums, super enhanced by the tipple!

"Wrreeaahh."

"AAAAAAAAAGGHH!"

I fell asleep easily, in a bottom bunk with Alan above. Too drunk to hear anything. Instantly zonked.

At around 3am I woke to a dripping, piss-smelling condensation gathering on the fiberglass base of the bunk above, dripping on my forehead and soaking my sleeping bag. Everything smelled of urine – did Alan piss himself? Actually, no. It came from obvious sources; the 'lads.'

"Wrreeaahh."

"Wrreeaahh."

"Wrreeaahh."

"Wrreeaahh."

I have never been so miserable. It would be comfier trying to sleep in a whale's rectum.

"AAAAAAAAAGGHH!" I said.

Aside from a brief interlude where I had to change a soiled pad, the next few hours were somewhere between sleep and conscious hell, freezing, damp, stinking mix of fag-end filled ashtrays, spilled whiskey, and bodily fluids. I was woken to the sound of Neil Young and sizzling bacon, there was a sharp sunlight focussing some warmth on my right forehead and for a moment I felt a good day ahead.

The light passed as soon as I got up to see it on deck, clouds and greyness swept overhead with a swift 'Fuck You.' Rain again.

Pitch Battle

I could hear mutterings from Alan, who was at the galley, fixing breakfast, and Bryce, who was audibly troubled with something. They had strong personalities, they were from the hospital in-crowd, 'The Boys'- actually. I was the relative 'boy,' they were fully grown hairy men. Bryce played in the hospital football team, as did I, but he was a moody midfielder, like a Roy Keane but less friendly. I played right back and hated that position, but it was a team of cliques, and I was the newbie.

I remember one game, where I turned up on a cold frosty morning feeling ill, a bit of a sore throat, bit of a cough, and just wanted to go back to bed. I remember telling Bryce, the captain, that I was feeling a bit ill – hoping maybe he would tell me to go home and look after myself, on the basis of there being enough subs. 'What? Are you fucking gay?' he sympathised.

It was only about twenty minutes in, and we were under attack (again), the opposition were up for it and I was being exposed, personally, I felt, due to the midfield, who all wanted to be scoring heroes, so they were always left up front complaining with their arms flapping about as they gave the ball away. The long ball came at me fast and very bouncy due to the frost. I jumped to get my head on it, flicking with a twist of neck to clear it to safety. Simultaneously, the opposition's big striker swung his fat size twelves with a full force shot, lacing it. Neither of us got the ball. I was smacked so hard in the face with his rock-solid, moulded studded, (cheap) Gola's, that I thought I had been shot. Lights out. Tinnitus.

As I was crawling on all fours, making my way off the pitch, dribbling blood, and dizzy, all I heard was Bryce shouting, 'Ha ha, you're fucking ill now you c*nt.'

Breakfast Baps

Bryce's groans and moans became shouty. Alan had obviously done something to upset him. It was something to do with a female they had both 'shagged' apparently. They sat opposite each other working through a bacon sandwich and shots of some kind of homebrew moonshine; great idea, I thought.

Then, without any kind of a warning, Bryce punched Alan square in the face. BOOOF!

For about two minutes there was silence, my jaw hit the floor as I prepared for an all-out fight in a narrow boat. I had time to map out my exit and even clocked the fire extinguisher that I would use to fire at them as if they were rabid dogs copulating.

Silence.

"Ooh, you shouldn't have done that Brycey, you shouldn't have done that," Alan repeated this a few more times whilst staring at him in a pre-explosive fashion. It was like a condensed 'Cuban missile crisis.' The tension was unbearable.

Nothing actually happened.

He got up and started packing. Bryce went back to his bunk, and I had understood the cue enough to help box everything up – obviously, the holiday had hit an abrupt end.

The silence mixed with relief lasted for hours, we

had to get the boat back to port, load up the minibus and drive for two hours. At any time or any moment, Alan was going to violently erupt.

Funnily enough, all the way home, I don't even remember a 'Wrreeaahh' or an 'AAAAAAAAAGGHH!' – they just knew.

In retrospect, and it wasn't really for me to question at the time, being a 'wet behind the ears' fresher, one could have called it. The overall impracticality of it all could have been pre-empted in a conversation that may have gone like this:

Alan to boss, "I'm thinking of taking some lads on a holiday."

Boss: "Great, where? And who?"

Alan: "Thinking of three lads from Block 6," (there were a wide variety of lads in the hospital, some, very able, with great personalities, and then there was Block 6. "Thinking of a Narrowboat trip."

Boss: "Er so you mean three profoundly handicapped, doubly incontinent wheelchair bound type of lads? On a Narrowboat?"

Big Al: "Yes."

Boss: "Erm don't you think that would be a bit impractical?"

Al: "How so?"

Boss: "Errrm, don't you think it may be a bit, erm, a bit too… um… narrow?"

The clue was in the name all along!

Never again will I find myself squashed in a vessel with two alcoholic psychopaths and three profoundly mentally and physically challenged lads. Bad dreams aside.

Becoming A Mental Nurse

Yes, I know, very funny! I would agree, most of the nurses turned out to be mental.

I got out before I became mental about fifteen years in, although some close to me may argue I was deluded to think that. Which, of course would indicate a dual diagnosis, unless they think my only mental illness was being delusional.

'Just because you are paranoid, it doesn't mean they're not out to get you.' A famous quote from some genius. Turns out, I do kinda think they are after me, but that is a whole other story.

Anyway, I started my three-year training a week after returning from my jolly narrowboat holiday.

It was confirmed pretty quickly that my need for an extra letter in my qualification did indeed mean I was likely to be working with a fair bit of faeces and dribble rather than people thinking they were hatstands. Never mind, my fellow cohorts seemed like a fun bunch. There were about ten of us and I was quickly drawn towards Andy who had a really great smile, he was also into the punk and reggae scene and liked to have a laugh, like me, often at the most inappropriate times, in lesson – we were big kids back at school in the back row.

This chapter will be fairly brief as not too much happened in the three years that has stuck in my memory banks. At the start we did a lot of biology and then learned about genetics and all the manifestations of 'disability,' syndromes, and defects – be it pre, peri or post-natal in origin. We learnt all the drugs and did a fair bit of general nursing.

From memory, we did something like six weeks in school, then a posting of three months on site learning the practicalities of what we had just been educated about. Some placements were in educational facilities for 'people with learning difficulties,' some would be in the institutional 'hospitals' with profound disabilities, some were in the community 'group homes,' then we did three months in general nursing; and then there were the secure facilities, with elements of mental illness.

I was drawn towards the group homes and the secure facilities, or forensic assessment and treatment centres. I liked to be able to have conversations with the 'service users,' do things with them like play football, and have a bit of banter (between fights).

One odd thing I remember was that we were taken to our placements by the most formal and elegant chauffeur! I have no idea why they didn't just send a battered old taxi or refund our bus fare. This guy was immaculate with a peaked cap that he would hold under his arm whilst standing to attention next to his immaculate car awaiting our arrival. I would like to say he saluted but I think that's one of those false memories one develops over years of embellishing an often-told story.

I would clock him whipping out a yellow duster to wipe and polish the most invisible blemish on his dark burgundy Rover 827 Vitesse. He would greet us with a "good morning, Sir," and drive us very slowly to our destination. I was happy with his slow driving as, in reality, I didn't want to go to where we were going! Sometimes I would try and make conversation, but his response was always something like, "Ah, well that's not for me to comment on Sir," – he was Parker out of Thunderbirds.

I can't imagine they exist these days. The modern version for the super-rich would be ex-military high performance drivers trained in tactical vehicular combat.

'Snot Fair

I was sent to my first day at an old farm building in the middle of nowhere that had been 'converted' into a group home for the 'subnormal,' pretty sure that's what the manager called them. He looked like a farmer. In fact, to be honest, I think they just swapped some cows for 'retarded' humans, probably much more profitable.

This was in the first days of 'care in the community.' They were closing the institutions as quickly as possible. The residents of such institutions were institutionalised, which was a bad thing, they said. So, the policy was to send them all back to their counties of origin and place them in 'community settings.' The trouble is the residents were 'institutionalised' – all they ever knew were the big 'bins' and, in the main, they were happy there. The vast 'outside community' was a big scary place whose inhabitants' pulled faces and called them names. I saw couples who had spent decades together cruelly separated and carted off to different ends of the country.

It seemed to me that it was quite easy to open a community home, and money was to be made. I knew of some colleagues in the bins who 'housed' a few in their attics and just worked from home – with a substantial pay rise – Cushty Rodney, Cushty!

This was a cold old farmhouse. This was where the residents had a morning shower that was literally a hose down in a semi-open shower block whilst lined up naked. To be fair, I think they separated the males from the females, I did the males. We are only talking about thirty odd years ago. I'm sure the authorities would have frowned upon it back then but receiving a 'frown' didn't really hurt.

Neither much of a deterrent or a punishment, is it?

My big memory from that place was on day one when I was being introduced to the residents. I was 'all smiles' and keen to show what a nice chap I was. They came up to me offering handshakes and seemed happy, in fact very likeable, and fun. Then Roger, a very tall excitable late teenager, came running up to me with the biggest dangling trail of snot you ever saw. He bashed into me with a massive cuddle and the entire green sticky thing wrapped itself around my face, across my mouth and down my neck. His breath was foul, old dribble being the top 'worst bodily fluid smell,' or a close runner up, in my opinion. You may be surprised to learn this if you've not experienced the full smorgasbord yourself. I pushed him off 'politely,' smiling on the one side of my mouth that I was prepared to move, to see an ever-growing connection between us like warm mozzarella. It was just horrendous. I don't want to remember any more from that place thanks.

Another least favourite placement was the block where Bryce's bondage partner was staff nurse. She was an uptight, a bit over the hill on a good day – Brighton

Drag Queen on a bad day, tart who liked to wield her authority at those who didn't fancy her. I didn't fancy her. She gave me the shit jobs. This was the unit with the most mentally and physically disabled, plus it was for those requiring some nursing, often bed bound and sick. She also didn't like me because I was somewhat attracted to another nurse and there was a lot of flirty banter going on, it didn't lead to anything, but it made the day exciting.

I remember having a talcum powder fight with her when we were either side of a bathroom divider. We had both bathed our 'patients' and had them on tables to dry and 'pad them up.' I started chucking handfuls of talc over the divide, often scoring a direct hit. She then went full blitzkrieg and thew over the entire box, it hit the top of the divide and disintegrated creating something like the largest snowball you could fashion, it landed smack on the face of my patient, who was still wet.

Although you won't believe me, I have to say the patient laughed and enjoyed the experience - just in case I'm reported 3five years down the line. He looked like the abominable snowman. I laughed until I choked. Explaining my 'accident' to the staff nurse, I could hear Sarah chuckling as she exited her cubicle. It took me ages to remove the caked mess from all orifices.

I decided to get her back by spraying a big cock on her car bonnet in shaving foam. Unfortunately for me, although it washed off, it had left a permanent lack of sheen due to the chemicals in the foam. Looked ok until a certain light hit it. Her Dad was furious, and I had to pay for a respray. Ooops.

I did some night shifts, which were double-edged swords. Generally, there wasn't much to do until the morning when you would start to change a few nappies until the day shift came in at 07:00. It was a massive, long bore though, there was no 24hr TV, no Internet etc, so you either needed a wordsearch book or allowed yourself to engage in conversation with the real night staff. The trouble with them is they are nocturnal and therefore have bugger all to talk about, they didn't do anything – apart from boring memories and photos of babies, they had nothing to offer – until someone had a birthday, then all hell broke loose.

It was the night matron's birthday, and I was informed that we would have a 'little get together' at midnight. Sounded awful. Slowly but surely the lounge area started to fill up with staff, and others from outside the hospital, someone fired up a ghetto blaster and drink was flowing. By 12:30 everyone was doing the Hokeypokey, empty bottles of gin and wine were replaced quickly by more. It was mayhem, people snogging on the floor rolling around in dog ends.

Then Bill Bonnet, hospital manager turned up. 'Holy fuck, we are all sacked,' I thought. His big red head broke into a massive grin as he revealed the two bottles of plonk behind his back, everyone whooped. It was clear he had already been on it for a good few hours, slurring and slapping arses like Sid James in a 'Carry On' film. Within minutes he jumped on to a table and started to gyrate, seconds later a leg collapsed, and he flew backwards, smashing onto the floor, clearly breaking his arm, it looked like a chicane. I was just gobsmacked. An ambulance carted him off while we all tried to clear up. The day shift arrived to find us all sound asleep to the ever-present odour mix of cigarettes, alcohol, and piss. 'Ah, it was matron's birthday last night, fair enough,' they said, jealously.

My only other memory of that unit was having to do a 'manual evacuation.' Sounds like fun, doesn't it? Like some kind of fire drill involving physical prowess or playing with a JCB. In fact, it is the delightful act of physically removing impacted shit out of someone's rectum. The patient was old, dying and in great discomfort. He hadn't passed faecal material for weeks, we (I) had to get it out. He died the next day. Luckily there is something in the hippocampus that somehow filters out the details of bad, explicit memory. For this reason, I can't give the details of tools and methods used and fully explain feelings of guilt the following day – all I know is, I did my best.

Meeting my mates in the pub that evening, we did the usual, 'what did you do today?' One had run a length of electric wiring around a house, another had delivered fifty pallets of pasties. I had dug a load of shit out of someone's arse.

The recruitment department of Mental Health Nursing really should employ me.

Forensic Gump

My penultimate placement during training was in General Nursing at the city general hospital. I really enjoyed it, it was very interesting, the patients were generally engaging and somewhat grateful. The medical science attracted me. Although I had to wear silly clothes, and I felt a bit gay (in the good old sense of the word, or is it? I dunno, for a punk drummer, I never thought I would end up being a nurse, it didn't seem very masculine). I started to think I had maybe chosen the wrong kind of nursing. There was a kind of chilled atmosphere, and female nurses' uniforms did wonders for my imagination.

Cue the secure forensic mental impairment / illness facilities. The bad boys.

The first odd thing was to be measured for my hospital suits; we were issued with a pair. Although not compulsory, they still issued the grey suits of institution. I only ever wore mine once (each), one for a wedding and another for a funeral.

This was the unit where Jeff worked, Jeff who caused me to collapse into unconsciousness.

On first sight it was very open prison like, with a secure wing.

The Brewers.

The Brewer family were all over the whole bin.

Big Mick was the Boss. He sat in his station, centrally

placed in the main living area of the unit. 'Walled' by plastic glass on all sides. He could see everything under his command. All you needed from him was the slightest of eyebrow movement and you knew if you were doing ok, or not. You didn't want to get on the wrong side of big Mick. He Bad.

His Sister, Brenda was a battle-axe in a matron's outfit, she ran pretty much the other half of the hospital, you didn't want to piss her off. She had her minions who also acted hard. They all stank of fags and brandy. I'm sure she had a nice side (once). There were sons and daughters and sons and daughters-in-law, cousins, and married cousins – probably from the same Norfolk hamlet. You really had to watch your tongue otherwise you would soon find out a 'little bird told them you'd been slagging them off' – Big Mick would 'clock you' as you walked past, and you would worry all day.

That's if you could see him. The station was in a permanent fog of roll-up smoke. He would be rolling one as he puffed on the current one. He would hold betwixt three fingers and a thumb with the lit end facing his palm, like a proper rock-hard east end thug. His eyes would do a Clint Eastwood as he took a drag. He was big and strong, very clean shaven and seemed to do fuck all except give 'looks.'

He was a charge nurse, that usually meant you trained to the level of staff nurse and worked your way up. I doubt if he did one day of training and suspect he achieved his status by default, having outlived everyone else. There was another level, known as Enrolled Nurse (EN). There were quite a few in the hospital, one being Big Mick's Mini-Me, Kevin – or 'Medium Kev' - had the same smart look, clean shaven, used the same phrases, always lit a fag when Big Mick did, squinted on inhalation, and sat in Big Mick's chair when it was vacant, despite trying (I am sure with several run throughs in the mirror), he just couldn't get the eyebrows to speak. It just looked like he was secretly farting. EN's were replaced by a new educational standard, NVQ – some of us thought this must stand for Not Very Qualified.

I was lucky to be allocated this unit because it provided the admissions and assessment phase of the forensic psychiatric service – so before treatment and rehabilitation. We really didn't know who we were dealing with until they came to us. It was exciting, interesting and a very macho environment, the females who worked there were also macho, think 'Prisoner Cell Block H.' You could get in Big Mick's good books without licking his arse (Eeew), if he saw you had some balls. Luckily for me I always got on with him, I didn't try - unlike Medium Kev, who tried so hard but never really got there. Bless.

I was offered a place on the full 'Control and Restraint' course, which lasted ten days and meant that I would be equipped and qualified to be part of an emergency three-man C&R team to deal with any violence – anywhere in the hospital. It all felt very SWAT.

Control And A Little Restraint

I don't think I've had so much fun as during this week and a bit.

We were doing the full course and that involved Shield and Riot Gear training AND we had a whole, recently closed, hospital wing to use as a battle scene. It was like being given a portal to step right into Mortal Kombat. The timing was epic.

We would learn the same techniques they use in prisons, policing, and by close-protection operatives, how useful I thought. If ever I'm being restrained in a riot, I would know their next move!

It was designed to teach the correct 'use of force' techniques, with non-compliant and violent individuals, who could also be armed with anything, other than a gun - within government guidelines of course.

The first half included some conflict resolution methods but mainly it was straight into the physical, initially learning breakaway moves and techniques to get out of strangleholds (a swift cricket bowling action with a 180-degree turn), hair grabs (a two-handed push down on the assailants' fist and a swift body drop) and bearhugs (heel down the assailants' shin and drop) etc. Don't try any of these based on the descriptions! Added to those is the twist-pinching of highly sensitive areas of skin – I can tell you now the techniques hurt like hell, get them right and your assailant will recoil, immediately letting go - wanting their Mummy.

However, and I've been on a few refreshers, people always go through the motions in practice. You team up with a colleague, one grabs the other and then they let go all too quickly once the defensive move is triggered. It is never like that in a real setting, generally the assailant is pumped full of aggressive adrenaline and/or drugs, they are mentally possessed, and they want to kill you, they ain't going to just let go because you pinched their 'bingo wings.' You really have to do it right and several times over, very hard and often slipping outside of government guidelines if you need.

If you are assaulted, it's best to get away as soon as you can. If someone is in danger due to a violent aggressor you need to 'take the aggressor down' as soon as possible, we would often say 'deck him' as the cue. Often, though you would not want to afford them the politeness of a warning, but you need a very well-coordinated team of at least three C&R trained individuals otherwise it can go horribly wrong. You also need somewhere secure to take the individual. It is possible to 'deck' and restrain a person by yourself, but you need an exit plan as I found out once on an outing with a small group of patients.

I had just qualified and went out to the local shops with three 'benign' patients (no history of aggression) and a nearly retired nursing assistant lady, who was the mother figure of the unit, unlike the other females. We were in a toy shop having a look around when I noticed this particular patient stuffing his pockets with various small items. He wasn't a likeable character but was never any real bother. I went up to him, leaned into his ear and shouty whispered, "What do you think you're doing, put them back. Now." Without warning he punched me really hard right on the nose, it was a great punch to be fair, no chance of me getting any guard up. So, I decked him. I had him face down on the floor in an arm lock whilst trying to clear the tears in my eyes (nose punches do that, I wasn't crying, honest). Pat, my colleague was horrified, as were the shop staff.

The trouble was knowing what to do next. I couldn't sit on him forever. I had to get him back to the unit. I could have called the police, but to be honest, I had only just started work in a management capacity and that would have looked like a pathetic failure. He was still threatening to hit me and was trying to do exactly that each time I relaxed my grip on him. So, we just stayed there for about twenty minutes, I explained to any passer-by that all was under control, and we were from the local mental hospital. He eventually calmed and I pretended I was just fine about being punched, "No problem, mate, everything's just fine and dandy, let's go back and have some cake." We got back into the unit, shut the door behind us and he was marched straight into 'seclusion' for a 'debrief' – don't read too much into that, all was within Government guidelines. No cake.

I checked in on him through the seclusion window after ten minutes or so, he came up to the glass and gave me the finger. I just smiled and I took a big, long bite into my wedge of Black Forest gateaux.

So, controlling and restraining a violent person requires an exit plan. We learnt how to safely remove a non-compliant aggressor and place them in a seclusion 'cell' – they were never 'padded' but there were no sharp edges or corners. It took three people, at least, and, if possible, a fourth – 'the head man,' not that they were the boss, but they controlled the aggressor's head.

The main tool for restraint is an arm lock. The main tool to deck someone is in the initial stages of that same arm lock. It involves rotating, extending, and then flexing the wrist and arm in a plane of movement that is counter to normal joint positioning, it makes the recipient have to recruit rarely used, weak, muscles to try and release themselves. You can hold the arm in such a position as to force them onto the ground with an extended arm or follow through into flexed joints to create the arm lock. A gentle flex of their wrist creates a lot of pain if they try to force against you.

If you are aiming to relocate the person into a seclusion cell, or a police van, you will need a man (or woman, obvs) on each arm. The third person will push the unwilling participant's head downwards so they are bent forward having a good close look at their own knees – then the four can walk in unison – like an overcrowded pantomime horse.

The fourth man isn't really required until you get the individual face down on the cell floor, facing away from the door, where they would protect the head from either self-injury, or biting, or spitting. You can also imagine a fourth team member being very helpful opening doors and clearing passages on the way to your secure destination. Many an operation has been scuppered by an unseen obstacle.

If you are only three, the head is free to go wild for the moments it takes to 'wrap them up.' This is the fun part. This is best explained in sequential bullet points.

- The three (or four) members have numbers, 1 right arm, 2 left arm, 3 legs, (4 head) – let's call the restrainee 'X'.

- You need to have X lying face down in the seclusion room / cell. They may not comply; in which case you need to trip them over in a controlled manner.

- The third member of the team (number 3) folds one leg so the ankle crosses the other leg at the knee in a figure 4.

- The long leg is then flexed at that knee and the foot pushed up towards the rear pelvis, thus

- trapping the other ankle in the crease of the knee.
- The number 3 guy places their own knee on the outer knee of the first folded leg and leans over the back of X, pushing their (X) other leg down by their (number 3) chest... You following? Yeah, I know.
- Both number 1 and number 2 have rotated X's arms back behind their (X's) scapulae, with both hands (X's) held together like little butterfly wings.
- Then, as number 3 is leaning over X, using their weight, they (3) hold onto both hands (X's).
- When number 1 is sure number 3 has a secure hold, they (1) run out of the room shouting, 'One Out'.
- Then number 2 does the same, 'Two Out,' if there was a 4, they would do the same – 'Four Out'.
- This then leaves number 3 atop of a grenade about to explode. Whilst number 4 grabs the back collar of number 3, 3 can spring down on all four limbs of X to bounce up and backwards exit, without dignity, quickly enough for the door to be slammed shut before they can be grabbed – by X.
- Bang! Job Done! Simple, isn't it?

DR CHRISTOPHER FORD

The final few moves are fraught with risk and precise co-ordination essential. You all need to exit the seclusion room, after letting go, slamming the door shut behind you before the wildly pissed off and dangerous animal gets to attack you – trust me this is their only aim in life at this point. Get it wrong and you're in big trouble. If 1 or 2 exit without 3 having a proper handhold, it all falls apart. If 3 doesn't get grabbed or their spring action causes them to fall sideways, they are toast.

The worst event, and it has happened on more than one occasion in my experience, is when someone gets over excited and slams the door shut with #'s 2, 3, or 4 still inside. If it's 1 you have seriously fucked up.

Call an ambulance!

We practiced restraining and secluding several times over, taking it in turn to be the violent nutter – which was great fun. As mentioned before, I just didn't go 100% because, in reality, I knew I could have just punched any one of them hard enough to make them go off sick and miss the rest of the course, especially (but not exclusively) some of the females.

That's all well and good but what if you have two nutters trying to kill each other? I mean you could just watch and take bets, which is what they probably do in Columbia, I'm guessing. We, however, have a duty to protect the individuals from causing either harm to themselves, or others, so both boxes are ticked. Obviously, if it takes a minimum of three C&R trained individuals to deal with one aggressor, you need at least six for two. As said before, in the real world, you never had that many team members on shift, maybe you could muster six from other units if they answered the phone! They did issue bleepers once technology allowed, and alarm systems eventually. Patients often hit the buttons for a laugh creating that inevitable 'cry wolf' response.

We had a patient in another clinic I worked in a few years later who's only challenging behaviour that led to him being in a forensic setting was setting off alarms. He had created merry hell for years, just couldn't resist it. I must admit to suffering the same impulsion – that emergency stop lever on a train, I have to avert my gaze. It was the fire alarms he liked the best because that brought out the big red lorries. Sirens and blue lights, what power he had. Being a simpleton, he called them 'Thyre Alarms,' "I'm going to sshmaf the thyre alarms," he would threaten before being carted off to seclusion. His problem was his other compulsion, which was to tell us before doing so.

The best bit about simulating the two-person fight was, you had to have a fight. To make it realistic, and tricky for the team, you needed to be grappling on the floor shouting obscenities at each other, rolling around trying to wrestle and 'soft punch.' My fighting partner was one Jeff James. How he laughed as we were calling each other 'Fucking Cunts,' 'Twats' and 'Wankers,' while slapping each other

– one of us wasn't acting.

Surprising fact: If you find one fighter on top of the other, you can lift them off and decouple him backwards using just one finger wedged hard up under their nose, it has that same paralysing, but momentary, affect cats display when dangled by the scruff of the neck.

So now the real fun bit. Helmets, Shields, and Riot Gear. The armed and dangerous 'psycho on the loose' scenario. It was time to learn how to isolate, disarm, restrain, and remove, while fully covered in awkward SWAT 'clobber.' To simulate this, we had about an acre of battlefield containing several buildings full of furniture, and untold miscellaneous items you would expect to find in a hospital. The whole lot was decommissioned and ready for demolition – we were allowed to smash anything up with whatever force and whichever implements we could lay our hands on.

It was the ultimate Hide-And-Seek! It went like this; you are the nutter, you have ten minutes to hide, arm yourself crazy, build up an arsenal of weapons and ammo, maybe a few stashes, and then, "We're coming ready or not." 'We,' being three or four fully protected shield holding predators coming to get you; they would get you one way or other, you knew that. But you would go out in a blaze of glory. I was the Sundance Kid.

The C&R team adopted the centurion formation,

number 1 holding the shield facing forwards. The shields were around three feet high and two feet wide, made from very strong clear plastic, you needed to be able to see through them, or hide behind to fend off projectiles. Numbers 2 and 3 would provide flank cover, one arm holding number 1 the other facing their shields outwards on each side. Number 4, if you had one, protected above and the rear – if you were stupid enough to allow the crazy killer access to your rear end! Ideally the centurions would resemble the Horseshoe Crab, impenetrable on top and sides - but with a bunch of wild flailing legs in its vulnerable underbelly.

The aim was to eventually back you into a corner, against a wall, taking all the slings, arrows and blows from the nail headed club, until you get compressed like a swatted fly, face all flat, white ischemic patches contacting on the clear Perspex shield that number 1 has kindly offered up – with the force of four over-excited hunters.

Just to let you know, if you are ever wielding a weapon at a group of riot shields in a mental hospital, they will take your blow and then advance one step as you pull your weaponed arm back to try your next hit. It only ends up with you going one step forward and two back. Once you are splattered against the wall, you can't move anything, number 2 or 3 will prise away your weapon and they will then armlock you while discarding their shields –

probably head butting you with their helmets at the same time, accidentally of course. Then you get wrapped up, Haloperidol jab in the buttock, and your day is done.

This twenty-minute rampage was probably the most exhilarating in my life. I was given ten to hide and tool up. Running without any direction, plan, or knowledge of the area, I found myself in a ward setting, hospital beds, trolleys, filing cabinets, chairs – utterly spoilt for choice. Working my way down corridors, I found a maintenance store, and in it, a long chunky pickaxe handle, perfect! Running back looking for a hiding place and more potential ammunition, I found myself in the toilets. You don't want to be 'caught and processed' anywhere near there. However, I thought chunks of porcelain from the 'Armitage Shanks' sinks would be heavy, sharp, and scary for my pursuers. I smashed them all up and quickly build up a couple of piles, pushing them by foot towards the entrance where I could see the open ward and all access points into it. They were coming.

Yucca plants make excellent projectiles if suitably hydrated. They have long 'holding-stems' and a heavy pottery base, you could use full hammer throwing technique if coordination and spatial awareness allowed, the gyrations would add to the drama of impending doom for the prey. I had six lined up. My plan was to wait for them to approach and just bombard them with a torrent of ballistics. Shock and Awe. I would be George Bush, and they Iraq. Then I would run, somewhere.

I saw them shuffling along, three men and a burly beefcake of a lady. They were shitting themselves. Clinging tightly to each other. Eyes darting in all directions, usually in pairs, but not always. Their strides were uncoordinated, so as one stepped forward another had stopped, they were bunny-hopping like a teenage learner driver. I waited quietly, heart pumping until they drew a bit further than level. I was very nearly behind them but felt sporting. At this point I let fly with a Yucca. It was a single-handed discus technique, the 'succulent' was dried and brittle, having sat there ignored for months, it snapped halfway through the swing but luckily the heavy potted base flew hard, flat, and fast, hitting number 2 right on the helmet. They all rocked, and I heard a girl scream (Jeff). Nobody was hurt. They stopped and heads turned my way. They were like an oil tanker in agility when it came to changing direction of travel, gotta maintain protection, rotate as one without leaving cracks in the shield cover.

"This way."

"No, this way."

"Go back."

"No, circle round this way."

"Wait."

"You step right, I'll go left."

"For fuck's sake!"

Blind leading the deaf, dumb, and blind.

Too late, I pelted them with ceramics and Yucca pots, whilst getting ready to 'leg it.' I was out of ammo, bar a few in the hand, as I ran across the ward and through a door. It had no exit. Damn I knew I was done for. They were getting close to the entrance I had just used, there was nothing in the room, just a bed. I had one option other than to activate my explosive suicide vest (which I didn't have). I grabbed the mattress from the bed and held it flat in front of me like a massive heavily stained shield… and charged at them. British Bulldogs.

They went flying, once one fell, they all fell. It was pathetic. I jumped over them, planting a foot on someone's back and trampolined through the only door and out. I won. As I ran, laughing hysterically, the C&R trainers pointed me to their left. I ran as directed. Bugger, an empty room. Leave the windows they said. I knew what was coming even though I still had the long wooden handle.

In they came, boy did they look vengeful. It was quick. I managed to strike them around three times, bash, push back, bash, push back, wall, no back swing, Gulp! Splat! To be fair, I was bloody knackered, once they disarmed, me using the twisted thumb technique, I was ready for decking. I got decked. I was wrapped up face down on some dusty lino – trying not to inhale dead and curled up woodlice. Restrained, lifted vertical, marched with my face pressed into my bollocks, and out to a round of applause. No Haloperidol unfortunately.

Coming The Counsellor

Back to Jeff, the inadvertent purveyor of priceless anecdotes (all given for free, as I said, price-less).

This big musclebound oaf created merry hell, the bull in the china shop. He was always the first to the scene of the accident, the centrepiece of any incident, as volatile as one of those spring-loaded suction pad toys. He would argue with his own reflection in Geordie quick speed. As subtle as a breeze block in your teeth. A compulsive pusher of buttons. The wind-up king. Once caught thumbing through a dictionary, "What are you doing Jeff?"

"I'm looking for *compassion* – don't know the meaning of the word." (not true, and a joke nicked from Alexei Sayle's great 'Didn't you kill my brother?')

Somehow, God knows, he became the unit 'counsellor' – a talking therapy involving a trained therapist listening and helping to find ways to deal with emotional issues, the calm space to share your most 'inner feelings,' a sanctity of upmost confidence and *compassion*.

How? How the hell did this happen? It's like using a pneumatic drill to ease a headache.

Apparently, he attended a course. I suggest a unit manager somewhere wanted a few days of peace, so they sent him packing on a kind of a pre-CPD training event, where, no doubt, he caused great disruption by constantly arguing with the trainer. Anyway, he made it very clear that he now had a certificate (of attendance), so we should all refer our patients (we had a key worker system so every patient had their first go-to staff member) to him so he could ease their troubled minds with his 'Nightingalesque' bedside manner. I believe some of us actually called him Florence, which he didn't 'get,' thinking it referred to a French rugby player.

Yup, that wasn't going to happen. We all saw how a few poor Guinea Pigs emerged from a session with him, it was if they worked for Pfizer. Didn't go well. In fact, they needed Counselling.

He would get very angry when nobody referred, it was always an option brought up in the Case Conference meetings (by him) that never quite got the vote. So angry that he went to the Unions about it complaining of victimisation in the workplace. He went to the Union (COHSE - The Confederation Of Health Service Employees – they left off the T otherwise they would be called 'Tea Cosy' which wouldn't be cool) on many occasions, always had a case against management for something. As said before, he wore a ripped-to-shreds suit for a couple of weeks because the hospital didn't readily provide him with a replacement following an ill-thought-out provocation with an armed psycho. He called the Unions in to sort it. It was always somebody else's fault and always a trip to see his Union rep. His Union rep would physically run away from him and hide. His union rep would be a different person every few months.

COHSE were always shouting about something, always up in arms, I found a lot of them to be odious and disingenuous troublemakers – so I joined the RCN (Royal College of Nursing). Actually, I was a total snob in that respect – I was definitely better than them. This backfired one day when COHSE voted a flash strike and all my colleagues walked out, leaving me alone with thirty dangerous nutters. Luckily nothing happened and I could probably have called for help but had to do ten times the number of jobs I should have.

After he ran out of 'COHSE reps,' and couldn't find anyone to help him take legal action against his employers, he took legal action against COHSE!... and lost, probably because he was a massive twat.

In later years, working 'in the community,' I was assigned to a reformed character who wanted to 'give back' and become a counsellor, so they told me. I went to visit to see if I could help him with his new goal in life. Seemed a nice chap but unfortunately, tattooed across his forehead, it said, FUCK OFF YOU CUNT.

On that note, Jeff the counsellor was often asked for his professional opinion, being an 'Enrolled Nurse.' That was our job, whatever level of qualification. We were in an admissions unit for the evaluation and assessment of people with mental disorders. Assessment, being an appraisal, evaluation being a judgement, we collectively arrived at a diagnosis, or diagnoses. The consultant was entirely reliant on our observations and conclusions, and for that we relied on our training and experience. Our opinions counted, and literally determined the futures of the individuals we 'cared for.' The inverted commas highlight the fact that some of these individuals did some nasty things – but we had a professional duty to rise above any feelings from the gut. Someone had to provide care for them.

We often had one-to-one interactions with our patients and were always looking out for signs and symptoms of mental disorders. Surely Mental Health EN's had some training in this area? I was used to picking up Asperger's traits, or signs of delusional psychosis, depression, PTSD, OCD, personality disorder, addiction, the list goes on. Jeff, the counsellor, obviously put himself right in the driving seat for picking up such traits, we relied on his insight and feedback. Usefully, his, 'by- far-most-often' diagnosis was… wait for it… "He's just coming the cunt."

'Coming the Cunt?' None of us had ever heard of such a syndrome. Apparently, it meant there was no disorder, the individual was just a difficult person. Apart from that possibly being a correct assessment in 1% of cases, I'd never, ever heard anyone else ever using such an expression, before, during, or after my life in the mental health business. Jeff James was one of those visionaries, able to define a particular subsection of behaviour, so specific that it warrants his name to be forever attached.

James's Syndrome (*A collection of signs and symptoms that can be classified as typically 'Coming the Cunt'*)

More on him to come. Sorry.

Chemical Castration

You may hear the term 'Chemical Castration' and imagine some kind of medieval torture procedure involving forced restraint and acid fuming testicles. In fact, it's not, it's just medication that reduces sex drive. Anaphrodisiac drugs, not even sterilisation, just some tablets that reduce libido – used with paedophiliac sex offenders. A temporary fix.

In our admissions and assessment unit, we also had some unsavoury characters placed with us long- term, they were a risk to society. We had seclusion facilities but were not a fully secure unit – inmates could escape quite easily. We had to keep watch on a couple of individuals who had a history of 'kiddie fiddling.' One, let's call him 'Bob,' had been there for many years before I arrived. He was an abnormally big man, a degree of 'learning disability,' but I think he also had some brain damage from a childhood accident. Everything about him was big, ears, lips, forehead, torso and occasionally you would catch sight of him naked if you were very unlucky. Everything was big. He did nothing all day except sit and smoke unless he 'kicked off' due to some random annoyance and then he would sit and not smoke in seclusion.

He would often break down in tears and explained the insight he had into his 'problem' – which were the intrusive thoughts about young girls. He wished he didn't have them, but he did. Looking back, I am struggling to work out why a sex offender would be in a semi-secure unit, if they required chemical castration. It clearly wasn't 100% effective because Bob kept getting urges. However, to my recollection, he never absconded, probably because he couldn't move faster than half a mile per hour and the unit was fairly isolated – it was surrounded by a few hectares of open land.

Nevertheless, he was often consumed with 'thoughts,' and that 'troubled' him somewhat. It 'troubled' me also. His room was upstairs off the dormitory – being a long-standing guest, somehow, he deserved a room. We always had the opportunity to peer in through the window in the door, which is when you may have unfortunately caught sight of a naked Bob, sometimes furiously 'mock-masturbating' as a show, especially for you. Nice. Privacy wasn't a thing there though, so we could also enter the room at any time to check for banned items, such as knives and drugs. We forced a strict tidiness and cleanliness regime as far as we could.

One of our student nurses first mentioned the smell. She said it was like vinegar but also a bit 'Scampi Fries.' I guess the rest of us were used to it, a bit like not really noticing your child growing taller until someone fresh comes in, not seeing them for a while, remarking on how tall they have suddenly become. The smell developed into a stench and after a week or so, we all noticed it. It seemed to come from the corner of the building, upstairs near Bob's room. But sometimes it travelled. It didn't go away. Our Polish janitor attempted to clean everywhere near what we thought was the source, he always had a fag in his mouth so a mixture of bleach and tobacco should have done the job – but it didn't. Had someone hidden an open tin of pilchards somewhere? Was a prawn sandwich wedged down the back of a sofa? Nope. It got worse.

One morning an unfortunate staff member walked past Bob's room, hand-over-nose, glanced through his door and thought they noticed something odd. It was so odd that they didn't mention it for a couple of days until we were having a chat over coffee. "Yeah, I saw Bob the other day hobbling around his room, no bloody clothes on again; and he stank."

"Sounds like him," I said.

"Why are his balls black?" he said.

"What?" said I.

"I don't normally look at another man's bollocks, but they are jet black and stick out at weird angles," he said, while dunking his Rich Tea biscuit. It was a bit of a conversation-stopper, I was lost for words.

At this point I was a Staff Nurse, second in charge to the 'Charge Nurse,' Mick Brewer. I told Mick Brewer, who was not one for leaving his central station, and Mick Brewer gave me the job of going upstairs to inspect Bob's balls. Some people lay bricks, I'm a testicle inspector, that's what makes the world go round.

He seemed quite happy to show me. The stench was unimaginable, I did it whilst holding my breath.

They were small, jet-black prunes. Pointing in odd directions, he walked in such a way you would if your bollocks were out of place. Then I saw something else that forced a sharp intake of breath - distressingly emetic. Rubber bands were tightly wrapped around the upper part of the scrotum, six of them, completely shutting off any blood supply to the testicles. The testicles were necrotic. Dead. Stinking.

He had actually castrated himself!

Three days later he came back from hospital minus a pair of bollocks. He was happy, unlike us who had to change the dressing twice a day.

One needed to adopt a limbo position while working upwards on the wound while he stood straddling, and conveniently holding his penis out of the way. Think of a mechanic on his back supported by a mechanics trolley, patching up the exhaust under a '57 Chevy.

This wasn't a 'Chevy', and it wasn't an exhaust pipe.

Still, 'one less paedo,' we opined.

Smith's, the 'Snack-Food Company,' lost a loyal customer that day, I used to love their Scampi Fries.

Penile Plethysmographist

I bet he never dreamed of this as a career when young.

The Penile Plethysmographist at Broadmoor Hospital, what a job. What number of notorious inmates' penises has this man prepared for Plethysmography, wiring, and strapping them up?

Of course, that wasn't his title, he was the Head Psychologist, running the brand-new psychology department at Broadmoor. They had everything purpose built, and we had to take one of our 'persons attracted to minors' there - the new 'normalisation term' our twisted governments seem hell bent on, they obviously think it's kinda ok these days to entice children into an unexpected experience of sexual assault with a fat bearded old man (probably in lipstick and heels).

Anyway… Jake, a nursing assistant and I picked up the hospital van and placed our paedophile in the back seat ready to drive the 178 miles to Bracknell Forest, a good three hours away. I say Paedophile but bear in mind that the purpose of the journey was to find out if he actually was one, and if he was, what flavour did he like? We had a good idea that this chap was one because his repeated crimes were dressing up in a white lab coat (with a toy stethoscope) pretending to be the school doctor in primary schools. The fact that he was fat and four foot high, with three teeth at best and resembled a gargoyle – maybe I'm being harsh on gargoyles – didn't seem to put him off. He often told me he was such a good-looking boy, and a 'beeeyoootiful baybee' - so delusional that he obviously thought he could pull it off. Queues of children offering close inspection of their private areas, no doubt. I think he rarely got more than a few paces past the front door, but I do know he was caught with children in other incidences. His name was Martin. Martin was not likeable, but we were professionals and we wanted to help him get through life one way or another. Martin was annoyingly happy most of the time. Three hours with him in a van was like sitting through a seventies end-of-pier comedy show, you'll like it, not a lot! Not at all.

We eventually pulled up to the security gates at Broadmoor, drove through the heavily reinforced steel entrance, through the big arched 'portcullis' type door between the towers and into the notorious hospital, everything was terracotta and grey. We were met by the Head of Psychology, who was as keen as mustard to show us their brand-new psychology department, recently opened, no expense spared, it was the 'gold standard' of psychiatric bin psychology facilities, 'state of the art,' they said. It was indeed a sight to behold, all clinical and new, shiny, and clean, black, and white, and chrome. A juxtaposition against the rest of the big old hospital. There were many computers and gadgets. At the time our unit had just had its first computer delivered and carefully installed, by a team in long coats, like it was mission control in Houston. I remember Big Mike, our charge nurse, looking and leaning over it, dropping fag ash on the integral keyboard, saying, "I don't trust these new-fangled compooders," he was such a visionary of things to come. This place had banks of them.

It also had a good old fashioned viewing gallery. For us it was entertainment, otherwise this was used for the educated detection of body language signals. Martin was now annoyingly excited as he realised all attention was going to be on him for the next hour or so. He was going to look at some pictures and they were probably going to give him some exciting sexual pleasure – as he was previously informed. I don't think he should have been primed, as that probably created unreliable results, a bit like studies only being single blind, or even with full twenty/twenty. Shame he wasn't given a nice surprise.

Jake and I were led away, Martin thought we were going to have some lunch, leaving them to it and to collect him later. In fact, we were quietly led up to the viewing gallery behind the large two-way mirror. Clever lighting and glass technology would mean we were totally out of sight. There must be no distractions for these things. We were in for a spectacular demonstration of cutting-edge clinical psychology.

The Penile Plethysmography measures the blood flow to the penis as a proxy measurement for sexual arousal.

It measures the circumference with something called an electromechanical 'strain gauge.' Alongside the 'strain gauge,' an airtight cylinder with an inflatable cuff was attached to the base of the penis. Maybe I'm odd but I think I would be turned on by just having such paraphernalia fitted.

As with a lie detector, there were other wires connected to measure sweat, pulse rate and I believe cameras that monitored where Martin focussed his eyes.

Then the show began.

This was in the days before HD porn movies were on tap to anyone with any kind of internet connection. It was the time when you still stumbled on wank mags in the bushes, if you happened to be there for any reason.

John and I could see the pictures that Martin was shown, they were done in short flashes. We were warned beforehand that they held some fairly explicit images for such purposes although one wondered how they actually obtained them – I guess from the police.

Most were benign, different people, different ages, different genders (there were just the two back then) but then there was a flash of something obviously paedophiliac. For reasons that don't need explaining, it was kind of awkward for myself and Jake – it's not as if we were rating them or pointing out the good ones. We just occasionally pulled faces like there was a bad smell or just looked away.

Anway, I guess we were about twenty minutes into the 'study' when Martin started to look around, he looked a little distracted, they must have been half-way through a batch of boring semi-clothed adults. He looked to the left, then the right, then up to air conditioning unit, then turned around and looked completely in our direction – at the large mirror. Him sitting there wired up with all kinds of contraptions attached to his cock, what a sight!

His face lit up. "Hello Chris, Hello Jake, what are you doing up there?" he said with a big grin, all thumbs up.

We spat our coffee out in an instant realisation that the 'gold standard' facilities were a bit shit. They didn't work – or somebody didn't set the controls right. I was as surprised as a duck coming in to land on water, only to find it was ice.

Martin actually thought we were all watching and enjoying the show! 'Great, isn't it?' I am sure Jake got himself into deeper water by giving a thumbs up back.

As far as I can recall, the rather expensive study proved 'inconclusive.'

The only 'outcome' was that Martin thought he, me and Jake had gone on a fun outing to watch a porn movie.

A Double Life

Like all of us working in those units, we had our demons, and our vices, guilty pleasures, and our escape shelters. Mine was smoking dope. I did it daily, sometimes the morning before a shift.

This proved to be an extremely bad idea when a pair of us shared a journey and a big fat spliff into work, we were on shift together, it was a beautiful sunny day. He was also the singer/guitarist in one of the bands I played in (The Whole Hog). We were super chilled, fobbed off the night staff with a 'don't bother' handover and started our day. Within moments, Adam, the same patient that subsequently strangled me with Jeff James on top, kicked off and started attacking another patient. My colleague, Dave and I got him into seclusion – not one of the cells but the seclusion lounge, where we thought we had sufficiently calmed him. We were a member of staff down so Dave went off to call for reinforcements, I saw him walking out of the unit with an unnaturally relaxed 'jive' gait. Why isn't he using the phone, I thought?

The next moment Adam went wild again and 'came at me' fists flying. I dashed for the exit. Dave, in his oblivion, had bloody locked it! I was locked in with mental Adam and I was wasted. Suddenly I was a wrestler fending off punches with cuddles, I had got him on the floor and was literally cuddling him with all limbs, holding on for dear life, keeping him decked and wrapped up. Where the fuck is Dave? I had sobered very quickly; adrenaline does override cannabis at some point. Though obviously not for Dave, a few minutes felt like forever, but he returned, walking nonchalantly with a colleague. I saw them laughing about something that Dave said. Naturally when they heard me shout, they became animated and 'heroically' sprang to my defence. Adam was strong – he once ripped the window out of a seclusion room, pulled the frame apart that had nails poking through, and started to flail it about like some kind of Celtic warrior. So, I was knackered and vowed (unsuccessfully) to never smoke dope on the way to work again.

I was also a drummer in a band – not that that is a vice in any way. It just meant that I mixed with all sorts of people. I was still a bit of a punk. At work, I was often in charge of my unit, and a key player with the psychiatrists and other disciplines offering clinical expertise. I was often chosen by the Consultant Psychiatrist to accompany him on assessments around the country to determine if prospective patients were suitable for admission. One such trip found me going to the police station in my local town where our band had played in a club the night before.

There were quite a few people there, we were all drinking together and popping out for a smoke. I spent some time having a chat and a laugh with a group that I didn't know too well although I had recognised from previous nights out and gigs. One seemingly nice guy was Dale, he liked his drugs especially the psychotics – mushrooms and acid.

It turned out that they had very much got the better of him as he had gone completely insane that night, hearing voices, seeing demons and both were telling him to kill – he hadn't, luckily, but seemed to have a good go at it.

The consultant and I entered the police station to assess this new patient, and of course, it was Dale.

I thought I was going to be rumbled, Dale was going to out me as a druggie in front of the consultant psychiatrist who shared great mutual respect with me. I was mortified. Luckily, Dale was totally fucked and didn't know himself let alone me. He was the zombie with the thousand-yard stare.

Phew.

He was subsequently sectioned, and we took him back to our place.

He suffered many months of absolute turmoil waiting for the antipsychotics to take effect, he became very fat in the face and body, almost seemed taller. As is usual, he took no care over his appearance, becoming the owner of a long straggly beard to suit his long straggly, oily hair.

Only a month or two before he was a healthy-looking young lad. It took me around four months to get a smile out of him, that was a little breakthrough and one of those few rewarding moments.

After six months or so he was well enough to do some work on the hospital farm, which he enjoyed. We also enjoyed each other's company, and, in many ways, I put more effort into helping him than the others. This was my duty as, for some reason Jeff Bloody James had it in for him. He would try and push his buttons.

You really didn't want to push Dale's buttons as he had become rather big and powerful due to the weight training that he had sought solace in.

Don't Look Back In Anger

Dale had also secured some 'parole' - meaning he could be escorted out of the hospital grounds for a few hundred yards (so backup could arrive promptly). This meant he could go to the petrol station shop opposite the entrance.

I think I mentioned at the beginning how, as a teenager, I would often be with mates in a car or on a bus driving past one of these big bins, how we laughed and mocked. One particular mock involved us screwing our faces into a 'mental patient' style, shouting 'Joey says, Joey says.' Some of you may already know exactly what that means and if so, you would now be well into your fifties and you would be British, having watched the BBC programme 'Blue Peter.' Either Peter Purvis, John Noakes, or Valerie Singleton would show us how to make shit things, like rockets out of washing up liquid bottles, whilst the presenters wore awful yellow polar necked jumpers and flared brown slacks. Sometimes John Noakes would do something daring, if he wasn't slipping up on baby elephant poo on the studio floor. It was a 'nice and English, and sensible,' Seventies programme designed to make us nice, happy, and compliant children.

They also thought we would like to know about Joey Deacon. Joey had, I believe, Cerebral Palsy, so he was all full of contorted and uncontrolled facial and bodily expressions and postures. He could only make noises, but he had a friend who could, remarkably, decipher them into meaningful words. His friend had a stutter. So, Joey would wobble about in front of Peter Purvis as he was being interviewed, Joey would then make all kinds of noises with more animated wobbles. Peter Purvis kept a straight face. Joeys friend then stuttered "Joey says, Joey says er, er, Joey says…" and then he would just make something up. Peter Purvis nodded like he was in a chat. It was a long drawn out 'conversation' that nobody understood. Obviously, a whole nation of early teens were pissing themselves laughing. What were they thinking? I remember being, very inappropriately, in tears. Next day at school everyone was running around going, 'Joey Says, Joey says.'

So, ignorant people often drove past making faces and noises, pointing up to the hospital blocks.

One day, I was with Dale in the Petrol Station shop (Dale still looked quite mental to be frank), we had just emerged into the forecourt, with our Mars Bars and Double Deckers, as a car drew up for petrol. Inside were excitable young men laughing. We could clearly see three of them in the back seat pointing and making noises. Then one of them turned towards Dale and, inexplicably, did the same thing! 'Digby, Digby,' he shouted. Where we lived, we used that term to describe a person with mental impairment. It was named after what was previously called The City of Exeter Lunatic Asylum in 1886.

'Digby,' he pointed, laughing with his mates. He suddenly stopped laughing when Dale punched straight through the rear window, grabbed his hair and parka hood, and proceeded to pull him back out through the shattered glass. Dale had become the Incredible Hulk - and looked like it.

For a nanosecond, I was bloody impressed and full of applause. But then sheer shock took over as a massive incident was obviously unfurling. The 'ex-laughing' boys screamed like they were being attacked by a T-Rex in Jurassic Park, the driver aborted his sweet shop stop, fired the ignition, and tried to drive off. I somehow managed to prise Dale's grip from the regretful fool and they got away, trailing glass, hair, and bits of coat as Dale and I flopped off their boot and onto the forecourt.

I radioed for help but managed to calm him before anyone arrived. Dale had a small cut on his knuckles but otherwise we were unscathed. I think we were both sitting on a grassy roadside verge having a smoke by the time they turned up. Laughing.

Busted!

Whilst I'm on the subject of Dale, I may as well bring old 'JJ' back in again.

Obviously, Dale lost his parole status – despite him heroically doing something that all movie goers would applaud. He was grounded and naturally rather pissed off with his lot. A good recipe for disaster is:

1. Take one disgruntled and once psychotic big man.
2. Add one ignoramus who thinks mental illness and depression = Coming the C*nt.
3. Mix them together in a small, contained unit.
4. Leave to prove.

The result is a volatile situation, a battle of wills, a fizzing time bomb. Both wound each other up. One of the two should have been professional enough to defuse, but this is Mr James (The Counsellor) – 'defusing ain't us,' should be his (ironic) catchphrase. They would bicker like an old pair of queens. Dale would call Jeff a Wanker and Jeff couldn't handle it – you can't seclude people for bad words, frustratingly. So, he had to get him back somehow.

One day Jeff arrived flush with excitement, "Oi, get in 'ere quick," he beckoned us staff. His face was beaming, eyes a little too wild, eyebrows elevated and alive, a bit out of breath… "I've got the bastard now," he declared.

We were all gripped with excitement and anticipation.

Actually, we weren't.

"I went through his drawers yesterday and found his stash of drugs. I knew he was on drugs, probably jacking up on that 'Marijana' in the toilets." He confusingly stated, like Joe Biden on a good day. "I found it though, and he is in big trouble, told you, he ain't ill, he's just a junkie, coming the cunt. You think he's mentally ill, but really, he's just snorting up some Ganja and probably supplying others."

"Where is it?" I asked, laughing inside at his ignorance, "show us then."

Jeff thought this was such a massive deal that he had proudly rushed it to the hospital managers office where he was informed that it would be sent to the Police.

"How much, what did it look like?" Jeff made a circle with his forefinger and thumb. "A big lump of that hash, weed, resin, you know, smack, a lump of dope."

"Does Dale know you found it?" I asked. "Nah, I'm going to let him sweat on it, go cold turkey."

For the next week or so we observed Dale – no writhing around the floor in pools of sweat. Nothing really any different. He didn't even look particularly bothered. I kept checking on him, asking if all was ok, I knew he had the odd puff and kept that between us, but he seemed his usual self, albeit still a bit pissed off.

The following week, it was Dales' Case Conference, we had the Consultant Psychiatrist there, the Psychology team, the Charge Nurse, myself, the OTs, and Jeff James – how he was present I don't know, maybe he said he had some information he wanted to share, or maybe he just wanted praise for busting the big drugs ring and had blagged his way in (offering counselling perhaps).

We discussed Dale's incident at the petrol station and decided he was provoked enough for it to be considered a behaviour 'somewhere within normal' parameters. Therefore, it wasn't a mental health relapse, or a sign of him being a particular danger to society. Anger management and COUNSELLING were discussed as a short-term response. Jeff's chair squeaked and quivered in excitement. We looked at the Psychologist who immediately confirmed she could do that and would fix up some sessions. Nobody could look Jeff's way, although we could hear him cough, sniff, and fidget. My eyes caught Dave's (The Charge Nurse) and we both knew to avert quickly before giggling. The last time we were all in the same meeting together, Jeff was pontificating about another patient, who's anti-epileptic medication was 'a waste of time' – because he 'never saw him convulsing on the floor' (in a full tonic-clonic seizure) – go figure! The bit that cracked us up (and you had to be there) was his pronunciation of Carbamazepine, otherwise known as Tegretol. Most people said Tegretol. Jeff wanted to go one step more scientific on this – *CAR-BA-MAZ-I-PEEN* – simple, try it a few times, CAR-BA-MAZ-I-PEEN. Just five simple syllables.

But old Jeff got to that part of his speech and stumbled out "KER-BAM-ZEY-PIME."

"Sorry?", said the Consultant, in a straight -faced request for confirmation, but really toying with his poor victim.

"KERBAMZEYPIME"

As I said, you had to be there, but Dave and I exploded, Dave was dribbling the chocolate that he was secretly chomping only seconds before.

We spoke about Dale's general behaviour and even agreed a slight reduction in his medication. We considered getting him more involved in the garden shop, and to interact with the public more - under supervision. As we were talking about his general behaviour, Jeff seemed at odds with everyone else when he piped up how erratic Dale seemed, how spaced out he was one minute, then wild and crazy another. Nobody else really agreed, we just moved onto another subject. We had all experienced JJ actually start fights in such case conferences by pushing buttons – the patients came in for the last ten minutes to have their say, and they would leave in a three-man team. We were leading up to that part.

The penultimate topic we moved onto, before Dale entered, was what JJ was looking forward to. It would imminently prove him right and us all very wrong. He would be the hero. The hospital manager had met with the police earlier that day and the police had the drugs report back from their forensic analysis department. The Consultant, who was the funniest guy you could wish to meet, once you knew him and once you understood his very dry wit, decided to read out the analysis report.

"I have an important forensic analysis report here from the Police, that bears some significance on today's meeting. Mr James may be keen to hear this".

Jeff sat bolt upright like he was at the Oscars.

"The results are in from the lab, and the readings are as follows: Cannabinoids 0%. Pebble 100%."

Cornish Daytripper

We had a nice old gentleman in our care, softly spoken, polite and nicely dressed. He was some kind of a tool maker in years gone by but was now retired and shared a home with his wife in deepest Cornwall. On the surface all seemed tranquil, pretty, and satisfyingly 'in order,' everything you would want in retirement, but apparently, one unremarkable morning he decided to greet her with an iron pan smashed across her innocent face.

He didn't have an explanation, no reason, no idea why. He just knew that he had done it. In fact, he called the ambulance to inform them. Quite calmly, no panic, which was very good of him. They needed precise location details and information about her current health – which wasn't great. She survived and he was quite pleased about that. He would talk about it as her 'having a unfortunate accident.' He was sectioned after a period in prison, I believe, and then he came to stay with us. He would call his wife every Sunday, as eventually allowed. He was taking some medication to suppress his 'personality disorder' and calmly worked his way through a year of virtual incarceration. He was a lovely, considerate, and helpful old man. He would eventually be returned to society and back home with his wife after a very controlled and carefully monitored 'deinstitutionalisation' process.

A defining moment in that process was to take him for

a closely escorted trip to visit his dear wife. She wanted him home and had come to terms with what had happened – although clearly concerned that it may happen again. We all were, to be honest. It was a two-hour journey, and I was not to leave him alone although I was also driving, so we weren't shackled. I was late up that morning and had missed breakfast but salivated at the chance to stuff my face in the staff canteen before we left, they did a mean brekkie including 'White Pudding,' which I loved; 'Black Pudding' not so much. I was starving.

"You'd better get off now, the traffic's bad," my boss said, handing me the keys. It was a Friday; everyone was driving down there for the bank holiday weekend. Damn, and bollocks, no big breakfast then. Frank, my charge, was smiling and smartly dressed, he had a bouquet of flowers. I wondered if an iron bar was secreted amongst the stems.

I couldn't stop thinking of sausages as I watched Frank in the mirror. He was happy and had a bright glint in his eye as he watched the countryside amble past. We were going slowly down a major dual carriageway; it was just past Eight in the morning, but traffic was building up. I was on the lookout for a service station, one that does sausages. My stomach ached with hunger, mainly because the thought of sausages set off my gastric juices prematurely, I was dissolving myself. I saw the sign, two miles to go – get in! We were supposed to get there by 10am because a social worker was going to arrive soon after to meet the couple, just in case all went well and he was discharged back into their care. For this reason, I declined the service station as it was also the centre of multiple queues of vehicles – everyone seemingly wanting fuel. Bank holiday traffic! The same twenty miles on, and again sixty miles on – all choked up. I didn't even need fuel, just sausages, but I couldn't jump ahead of the queue at the till just because of that. I did think about leaving Frank in the van and shouting my special need for 'emergency' queue hopping due to my unshackled and deranged criminal but decided it wouldn't wash for 'emergency sausages.' So, I bypassed them all with a heavy heart.

Frank and I spoke about how he met his wife fifty-two years before in the town five miles from where they lived. I don't think either had been outside of Cornwall, until Her Majesties courts pulled him out. I had convinced myself that the can of 'Lilt – with the totally tropical taste,' was feeding me. Surely his wife had some biscuits, I reassured myself. Let's just bloody get there.

I saw a roadside shop just after we passed the old village sign and was just about to pull over when Frank excitedly shouted, "There it is, Fuchsia Drive! I'm Home."

Bugger.

We pulled up next to his pebble dashed house. It was small and I could hear a yappy dog. Oh god, not a bloody Jack Russell, I thought as I remembered being bitten in the gonads by one several years before. It was called Cindy. We didn't like each other from the off.

Mary, Franks wife, was a little old housewife in a pinny and dirty slippers, her sleeves were rolled up like those wartime adverts. She had a few teeth missing. Not sure if that was Frank's dental work. Nice lady but talked too quickly and sounded like she was from darkest Norfolk rather than Cornwall but all these country-folk sound the same, to me. I was once in Arizona approaching the back end of a busy drinking hole in the middle of a desert, I could hear the chatter inside and was convinced they were all from Barnstaple.

Anyway, we were invited in after the longest hug in history, the last ten minutes was just unnecessary, a tad selfish I thought, considering my overriding hunger. As I was invited over the kitchen step Mary saw me notice the nice little pile of dog shit next to the fridge. "Oh, don't worry about that," she laughed, "it's normal."

Normal? For whom or what? I was quickly ushered into the lounge, which felt damp and muggy. The ornaments were of such bad taste I began to like them, like they were competing against each other. Lots of badly painted 'cute' smiling children with oversized tears on their cheeks – what the hell was that all about? And dogs in tartan clothing. On the wall, above the mantlepiece, which was above the electric 'flame effect' heater, there hung proudly was the famous print of dogs in clothing playing snooker and smoking pipes. The cheap plastic frame had come apart in one corner.

And then it came, talk of food!

"You hungry love? I've got some luncheon meat in specially." I imagined luncheon meat to be 'Spam' from a can, probably machine recovered soft tissue from the noses and lips of spent carcasses. Or maybe the Gabbernachulum. As an early teenager one of my friends told me that the bit of skin between one's scrotum and asshole was called the Gabbernachulum, and I neither questioned it or found an alternative (Perineum) until I was in my thirties. I believe I once told my doctor about my 'sore Gabbernachulum' after a vigorous bike ride – I thought his weird expression was a wince of empathy, obviously not.

I was also misinformed about luncheon meat. Clearly it differs from Spam as: *luncheon meat is made from a blend of 'meats' that are ground up and then shaped into a loaf, whereas Spam is made from chopped pork 'shoulder'* (Yeah Right) *that is combined with 'ham' and then canned. Also luncheon meat is sliced and served cold or at room temperature, while Spam is usually fried or grilled before being eaten – with thanks to Andrew Carter at MyConsciousEating.com (The Number One Source For All Foodies, Cooks, and Food Enthusiasts Around The World)*

Number One - for all Foodies, Cooks and Food

Enthusiasts! Anyone who eats basically. Number One!

I was bloody starving and would gobble it all up in seconds regardless of its status and content. It's always a bit off-putting when you can hear the chef preparing your food, cough and sniffle while intermittently over-stepping some dog shit – but I put that to the back of my mind and asked Frank about the ornaments.

"Ta Da!" went Mary as she entered the lounge with my plate full of sandwiches. "Wow," I said, "You're a star." For some reason, neither Frank nor Mary were eating, they just sat on the sofa holding hands, strangely with few words, other than, 'You alright love?' and, 'Yeah.'

I launched straight in.

Immediately, I was aware of some strange textures, fibres, tickly sensations on my soft palate. It took a while to retrieve them from the back of my throat to the accessible front with my tongue. They would stick. I had to make those odd throaty sounds you hear in harsh Arabic languages. I grabbed what I could feel and pulled it out from my mouth.

Dog hair! Short white and brown arrows of Jack Russell body hair. On closer inspection they were everywhere, on the plate, stuck to the stupid bit of cucumber, all over the white sliced bread, and (curling up one side like a duvet for bed inspection), all over the Spam (It was definitely Spam). My meal was 26% dog hair. 70% Pig's lips. 4% Wheat.

"Um. Ooh, that journey, the traffic, phew the heat"

"I feel a little sick, bit nauseous. Best not eat for a while, let it settle," I said, unconvincingly, mouth still full.

Hunger can drive a man to kill. Maybe that's what triggered the Cast Iron Saucepan incident?

Anyhow, I needed to spit everything out quickly. "Can you show me to your bathroom, please?" Spoken with one bulging cheek. It was right next to the kitchen. I popped in, spat everything out and just stood there contemplating for a while.

We were expecting the Social Worker in around thirty minutes, so I had some time to sit with the couple, but I was feeling weak and shivery. I needed food, sugar, energy, urgently. They seemed to be happy, but I had no idea what was going through his mind, everything seemed calm, albeit in a grim setting. I was becoming overwhelmed with hunger and felt awful. I pretended to have a need to blow my nose, just so I could go to the safety of the bathroom again.

"You OK Frank?"

"Mary?"

"I think I've got a touch of hay fever, very itchy eyes, need to wash them," I said – my subconscious mind was telling me to stay there whilst it hatched a plan. That corner shop. Pasties. Crisps, Mars Bars. "I'm going to be a couple of minutes in here – need to rinse my eyes, I think it may be a dog allergy, you guys, ok?"

"Yes, my love, I'll put Cindy upstairs," said Mary.

I heard her go up, shut the door, and come back down into the lounge.

I bolted. Ran out of the kitchen, down the garden path, scratching my arms on the rose thorns, out of the gate, left, running like mad, past the bus stop, across the junction blindly, and jumped into the shop. Grabbed two pasties, a bag of crisps and three bars of chocolate. I threw a twenty-pound note at the old man, "Keep the change please thanks."

"Errr wait, hold on sir..." I heard him say as I exited, all the time I was thinking 'Please don't kill your wife Frank – please don't, please.' I ran like hell, dropping a Mars Bar, back into Fuchsia Drive, in through the gate, scratched my other arm on the roses, jumped into the kitchen and back into the bathroom.

"All ok you Guys?" I squeaked nervously through a wheeze. Silence.

"Yes, all good" said Frank after a few seconds.

"Mary, Mary, you good?" I shouted in panic.

"Yes love."

Thank fuck for that, I thought as I was choking on pasty. I grabbed a few big mouthfuls of chocolate and more pasty, before popping my head into the lounge to explain how my runny nose and watery eyes had now led to bloody arms. "I get these flare ups, allergy attacks, intense scratchy arms, I've drawn a bit of blood, it makes me a bit short of breath, a bit sweaty. Don't worry it's normal." I panted, quite proud of myself for explaining the blood, sweat and heavy breathing, all in one go. I even got her back with the absurdity of what is 'normal.'

They obviously thought I was falling apart, I cared not, I had excuses for several bathroom visits to fill my face from my overstuffed pockets. All was well. Frank hadn't splattered his wife's face with ironware, and my belly was full.

On our return, my boss asked me for the receipts for the lunch I would have bought so he could reimburse from 'petty cash.' We always maxed out our subsistence budget. Not I, but others, would add in some 'extras' for their dinner when back home. We always came back with receipts. "No need boss, his lovely wife made me an awesome slap-up meal."

Time To Move On

I was nearing the end of my time at this unit, in fact the whole hospital and geographical area. I had some personal issues with immediate family that, for the greater good, meant I needed to move away. I felt my young son was being affected by the constant 'arguing, toxic atmosphere, splitting up, getting back together' cycle, that his parents were creating. I needed to get away and nurture a healthy relationship with him, albeit from twenty miles away.

We had some pretty bad events at the unit before I moved, there were a couple of suicides, one a son of a rather famous person, and the other an angry young man who was soft inside, simply looking for direction. I was the 'primary nurse' for both and very much liked them both. I always said that for most of our inpatients the most likely future for them is unintended drug overdose, suicide, or finding God and being taken in by the church. Although we were providing 'treatment' for a large percentage, and, therefore, there was some expectation to get them better and rehabilitate back into society, I didn't hold out much hope for them, this lot anyway. There was not much in their environment that felt 'therapeutic,' except maybe the farm.

The son of the famous person died soon after leaving us so, luckily for me, I was not involved but the other poor soul slashed his wrists in the medical room while waiting to see my colleague. He had somehow acquired some shavers and prised the blades out, saving them for what he felt was the right moment. He was found in a pool of blood; I saw the ambulance pulling out just as I was driving in to start my shift. As I entered, I saw my colleague in a fairly distressed state sifting her hands around the blood, which was becoming more viscous, as she was trying to find the blades.

FUCKING HELL, STOP! GET YOUR HANDS OUT OF THERE! This was during the time when AIDS was the big scare. She was literally wrist deep, with no gloves, wallowing around trying to feel and retrieve the sharp blades. Clearly, she was unable to think straight. I told her to go home, have a fag and a large drink, our form of counselling, or debrief. (Debriefs were introduced a few years later – for what they were worth).

The other horrible parting shot, before I left, was a nice young man murdering his Granny. He was psychotic, simply from smoking cannabis, hydroponics, but he smoked a lot. Maybe he did take more psychoactive drugs such as LSD, but I do not recall that to be the case. When he was calm, he was a nice, gentle lad with a pleasant smile. He never became violent but would 'disappear' into very deep, catatonic, silent moments, his eyes dilated black, face contorted with demons. I believe his 'sectionable' behaviour was a lot of murderous talk, voices telling him, encouraging him, it became a compulsion. He lived with his lovely grandmother who very much felt unsafe. I spoke with her several times on the phone, she really loved him but would often say how she worried how he may kill her if given the opportunity. After a short period of assessment with us, he was eventually moved on into a more secure unit. A few days before I left, I heard he had somehow travelled to Cornwall and killed her. The secure unit wasn't very secure, it seems.

I was asked, during a case conference, why I was leaving. I was going to a specialist unit near London which was supposedly the best in the country for forensic mental health 'evaluation'; they would take patients, with duel or multiple diagnoses, off their medication, in a controlled manner, and evaluate from scratch in the hope of formulating the most appropriate treatment plan for the most up-to-date and accurate diagnosis.

I told them I was going there because they fully evaluate, diagnose, and treat, or refer, and that appealed to me.

"Don't you think we do that here?" said the Consultant.

"Not really," I said. Unfairly, looking back, because the grass was definitely not greener, in fact, it turned out to be parched, with bare patches of cracked earth. Dandelions without the flowers.

The Original Asylum

Chaos, Pandemonium, Topsy-Turvydom, Booby hatch, Crazy house, Cuckoo's nest, Funny farm, Loony bin, Madhouse, Nut house, Sanatorium, Snake pit... Just a few of its synonyms.

Sticking to form, I'm not going to reveal exactly where I worked for obvious reasons but above is a clue.

As a staff nurse, I was allocated the best block of nursing accommodation, it was in grounds fitting for a king, beautiful lawns, and woodland. We had a lovely football pitch and a nice local pub. Everything you needed was in the local town or in London twenty minutes away.

I shared an old house with five or six others, we each had massive rooms that easily accommodated a double bed, lounge area, office area, loads of cupboards and shelving, windows on to sides and a handy sink to piss in when drunk.

I arrived in my black Mark III Capri full of hope and great expectations.

And that was my big mistake.

The black Capri, for some reason meant I was a wanker. There was a fully established clique in 'da house.' I was instantly not liked. For some reason they were all either Scousers or Scottish. The fact that I supported Liverpool made no impression. By this time, I had developed an assortment of insecurities, anxieties, and general neuroses. I would have panic attacks in supermarkets, or even talking face to face with someone. I would feel myself go bright red and sweat, then overcome with the urgent need to run away.

Smoking dope didn't help. Yes, I was a 'psychie nurse,' surely I knew that?! I had done it daily since I was fifteen, so it was a little more than a 'habit.'

They were complete twats though, very unwelcoming, in fact quite hostile. They would mess with my space in the fridge and often leave as a group when I entered the shared lounge.

One of them, a senior staff nurse, Scottish, very harsh accent, good looking but a complete bitch, was my initial line manager on my new unit, simply because she had been there longer – I imagine now she has long lost her looks and has those multiple branches of upper lip creases angry middle aged female smokers get, oh well.

She was the girlfriend of a Liverpudlian gobshite drug dealer, who also lived in the house, but wasn't an employee of the hospital. The first thing she got me to do was clean a toilet after a patient had been sick everywhere. My first day. I could only imagine how she laughed as she told her sycophantic housemates. It was a hard environment, I imagine like military barracks, you had to get through some shitty initiations before being accepted.

Pathetically, I was instantly accepted when the Liverpudlian, let's call him Dwayne, poked his head into my room as he could smell my spliff. "Wow man, you smoke weed." Everything suddenly changed – this was after three weeks or so. I had met some others who lived in a different block who I got along with instantly, so I was not miserable or lonely. I just thought they were ignorant fools.

They thought I was a wanker because I drove a Capri – simple as that. I was told that to be the case. I imagine a few wankers did drive Capris but surely also BMWs and Vauxhall's? Personally, I thought wankers drove Sierras.

Anyway, Capris were great fun, rear-wheel drive, so easily 'lost' on roundabouts, unless you were a speed drifter, like me. (I actually sound like a right wanker).

So, I was then suddenly accepted. I got on well with a couple of them eventually, in fact two turned out not to be twats. The others remained twats.

One of them used to stand too close to me when conversing, it was obviously a domination tactic. I met him years later randomly in a London street. He started to lean in again, so I stepped a little bit forward, and then I started to lean in. We had the most ridiculous close-face stand-off, while talking. He cracked first! Couldn't handle it, couldn't take his own medicine. Eyes started to flick left and right, couldn't hold his stare. Just like two boxers in their pants the day before a fight. He recoiled, nervously laughing. It was a small victory for the common man. I was surprised how I overcame my usual social anxiety; it gave me hope – albeit short lived.

Working in tough environments, your colleagues are piss-takers, cynical, cold, and unemotional. You had to be. You also had to be a hard drinker and a smoker. If you didn't go for your fag break with the others or the piss-up after shift, you became excluded. The women were rock hard. Those who stuck around for more than three months anyway.

Living in nurses' accommodation effectively meant you were at work 24/7, the nutters were spread equally amongst patients and staff. It was also one big knocking shop, which had its pros and cons, great for one's own needs, gossip and scandal, but often you would upset someone, either a jilted rock hard and angry female, or some bloke wanting to smash your face in. Luckily, I had my son, which meant I needed to travel away from it all fairly regularly.

My unit held around twenty-five patients, it was a secure environment, so they were all locked in. We supposedly had a high staff/patient ratio, enough for two three-man teams to deal with violence including more than one participant. Most of the time we were containing them but, during the day, various professionals would waltz in and see the nice side of the patients. They were often raising eyebrows when learning about the mayhem occurring in their absence. Clearly, they thought it was our mismanagement, but we really didn't have the Jeff

James's of that world. We were just the one's with the keys and the responsibility to say 'no,' so inevitably we were the ones who got it! We had far more incidences of violence than my previous unit. Partly because we took patients off their medication, and secondly, the design of the building had narrow corridors which seemed to compress the tense and volatile atmosphere, a bit like those films of Alcatraz, with the spitting inmates poking their heads through their door windows either side of the long dark corridors. You always had to pass someone in a dangerously agitated state. Once you passed three or four, you would also experience some kind of a werewolf transition.

Very quickly, I realised we were simply the jailors. The day visitors; the Psychologists, the Music Therapists, the Counsellors, the Voluntary helpers with chocolate, and the Consultant Psychiatrists (especially the Consultant Psychiatrists interestingly), got the best from our inmates, at least they were very rarely attacked. They all seemed to be of the same ilk, very lefty, all a bit 'right on,' coloured corduroy trousers, Save the Whale badges. Guardian readers. They did a lot of eyebrow communication with us, either raised or frowned, both had the same message. We would all be rather jolly with each other but there was a clear divide.

It was constant fighting, secluding, and filling out incident reports. Then they added the debrief sessions mentioned before. A counsellor from outside was brought in to help us 'understand' and 'make sense of' what we experienced the day before, most of us had forgotten by then having obliterated those memories with alcohol before they settled in the deep hippocampus. I am sure she had good intentions, but she just really annoyed us, having zero understanding of what it's like trying to keep the lid on a 'soon-to-be-exploding' pressure cooker. I guess the aim was to work out what went wrong when things went wrong. Someone always got hurt, but generally we were very good at containing aggression and dealing with it. We debriefed in the pub and usually laughed our tits off at it all.

Sometimes you just had to have a laugh and play pranks on each other.

You Can Hide But You Can't Run

One of our team was an Irish chap called Barry Ball – not his real name but it was yet another alliteration. Barry was a taker of the piss. He had a great laugh, one that would just make you want to join in without knowing why. He also had the most irritating patient assigned to his 'primary nurse' role. This patient, let's call him Geoffrey, went on and on, talking absolute rubbish, not entirely gibberish, but that of a three-year-old. "Are we there yet?" times thirty.

"Barry, Barry, when's tea? Barry, when is tea and what is it? When's tea did you say Barry?"

Geoffrey really looked up to Barry, Barry was the best. Geoffrey boosted Barry's ego, he liked to be held in such high esteem regardless of who it was from.

My 'most proud of' prank involved Barry and irritating Geoffrey. It happened by chance, as the best things in life often do.

Barry and I were in the staff room having a fag and coffee, catching a well-deserved break. I believe Barry was in the middle of a well-developed roasting at my expense, he was approaching the crescendo with great enthusiasm.

Our staff room policy was that we had to keep the door open to ensure a quick response to the panic alarms. Unfortunately, this meant most breaks were curtailed due to an incident or someone poking their head into the room simply to pester; the patients knew it was 'out of bounds' but that didn't stop them.

Anyway, Barry's glee was curtailed by the ever-increasing volume of Geoffrey's, "Barry, Barry, Barry, Barry."

"'Fucks' sake, fuck off," said Barry to himself and a chuckling me.

Then he had a brilliant idea.

Looking at me through his bottle-bottomed glasses and massive excited eyes, He put his finger to his pursed lips. "Shhhhhh, shhhhhhh, keep quiet, don't say anything," he said, as he dropped down on his knees and started to crawl behind the chair that I was sitting in, facing the door.

"Barry, Barry, Barry!" – it got louder as Geoffrey approached the door. Barry was all curled up behind me, hidden, trying to suppress his giggles.

"Shhhh," he reiterated.

Geoffrey poked his head in. "Barry, where's Barry?"

My brainwave came from God, it was so brilliant, and I continue to thank him for it to this day.

"Barry?" Said I.

"Not sure mate, shall we go and find him?"

"Actually Geoff, why not come and have a seat and I'll go and find him for you."

Geoffrey was made up, he was being invited into the staff room, and trusted to sit there alone, he knew this was not allowed, he instantly felt special.

"Yes, um OK Chris, thanks."

I stood up and gestured a welcoming arm to the inviting comfy seat.

"You relax mate, I'll go and find him."

This was the exact point where Barry could have saved himself, he had one chance but needed to think quick, like in a nanosecond.

He couldn't, his excited mind must have been slipping gears rapidly, signals must have been hit with sudden interference, what's happening? Houston, we have a problem.

Suddenly Geoffrey had sat his sizeable bulk down centimetres in front of Barry's little face, Barry stayed quiet, curled up awkwardly, and I left the room with a bang as I pulled the self-locking door shut.

I had won the world cup! Scored the winner! On cloud nine, and laughed like a crazy fool, OMG! Gotta go and tell everyone. Ha ha!

Five minutes later – which must have seemed like five hours for Barry – he came bolting down the corridor. "Bastard, you fecking bastard" (Still managing to say fecking instead of fucking, which was his self-imposed moral when in front of the patients, admirably.), Geoffrey was chasing him, "Barry, Barry... Barry!"

Barry had just endured a most painful period in his life, pure agony. His ego being crushed behind Geoffrey who was literally sat on top of him. Geoffrey was relaxed, king of the world, belched and muttered to himself, he may have even farted.

"You fecking bastard" Barry said again, with an incredulous grin, but the grin of a loser, still trying to come to terms with his unexpected period of angst, confusion, and turmoil. His funny plan had backfired spectacularly.

He waited behind Geoffrey for a few whole minutes, heard and smelt him, hoped for my swift return, which didn't happen, and endured a few more minutes trying to work out how to suddenly appear, how to crawl out from behind the chair in which the unsuspecting Geoffrey was reclined.

This was what he came up with.

"I got my pen out of my pocket, threw it on the ground near me, coughed, said, 'Ah, there it is – oh hello Geoff, been trying to find that pen, got it now, ok back to work,' and I just crawled then walked out quickly, not looking back, head down. That didn't just happen, that didn't just fucking happen".

It did, Baz, it did.

Vine Street Run

This, I believe was my most favourite of errands. For a while, I became a courier in London, driving around delivering stuff, pre-mobile phones, so no google maps. No, it was a case of fumbling through the good old A to Z, a London street map book. Surely road traffic accidents have plummeted since those days. It was impossible not to crash, while trying to find page 67, which was the immediate block of map to the East of page 21. My big crash was due to this, didn't quite stop at the junction, poked my nose into the main road crossing, just as a skip lorry whizzed by. My entire front end and bits of engine were suddenly strewn twenty yards down the road to my left.

Anyway, I digress.

My favourite errand was the 03:00 Vine Street Police Station Run. Basically, we just had to fetch something from the Police station and drive it back to the Regional Secure Unit, around five miles as the crow flies, ten as it walks, one hour by day, about twenty mins by night, flooring it. The item was one massive Jamaican musclebound man, in deep and wild psychosis. They had him in a custody cell like a caged wild stallion. He needed to be in a very secure mental unit. I believe several people were in hospital after he went batshit crazy with a pool cue.

I was doing my stint of night shifts; they were usually

DR CHRISTOPHER FORD

fairly uneventful. Patients were either asleep or locked in seclusion and sedated by midnight. Then the long drag through the small hours, as explained in an earlier chapter, awful TV, just two channels all night, no 'devices' (GOD I MISS THOSE DAYS), so you needed a good book or the ability to talk about things you had no interest in, usually just listening to your colleague talk about their dog. However, there was an awesome Turkish kebab takeaway in town that stayed open until 02:00 – someone somewhere could venture out for a break long enough to bring back several. I got fat there and then - and have struggled to 'not be fat' ever since. Damn those night kebabs… and chips (cheesy chips), and Mars bars. Crisps...

The Regional Secure Unit was as it sounds, highly secure, for dangerously mental individuals needing to be locked away. We had a large RSU next door to our unit. We were also secure but only one layer, so a locked reinforced wooden door (three if in seclusion), whereas the RSU had several layers of locked heavy metal doors, plus high fencing, and a security gate.

One night, the RSU was short staffed. That night came the call from Vine Street.

We needed four fully trained C&R (Control and Restraint) nurses plus an ambulance and Ayrton Senna.

Driving up there felt a little like being the SAS on their way to the Iranian Embassy, although we were only armed with vials of Haloperidol, syringes, and long deep intramuscular needles for big buttocks. And plastic cuffs.

The SAS obviously had flash grenades, machine guns, pistols, and body armour, so the jeopardy for us was far more serious (joking of course). I am actually writing this on the anniversary of that brilliant military operation, the storming of the embassy, full of armed Iranian terrorists, or was it the CIA? - who knows these days. Forty-four years ago, live on TV, Operation Nimrod – the SAS at their British best.

Anyway, ten years on, it was us. Planning our tactics, getting our kit in shape, writing goodbye letters to our loved ones. We made our way to central London. Professionals.

We were briefed on arrival.

"Eez in there. Fucking mental. Massive. Good luck, oh, and eez covered himself in piss."

Some patients are that often secluded that they know to cover themselves in oil or butter in preparation for the big restraint procedure. It worked very well. 'Hat's off.' It was like wrestling an Eel. It usually meant that you slipped awkwardly, kneeing them in the groin or other unfortunate areas.

No butter, or oil, but piss. Another old tactic.

This was pre-Taser days, so it took a van full of police, with batons, to get him into custody. So, there were four of us and around four coppers. The plan was for the Police to try and explain that we were here to help him and if he could politely move back into the corner, we would all come in, and gently help him out.

"Raaaaas Claaaat! Yooo Babylon Ting, Fuck Yoooo Boomba Claaaat Pig, I kill Yoooo Pussy Claaaat, Raaaas!"

In translation this meant, 'No Thank You Constable.'

All quickly agreed that negotiations were done. The Ambulance was waiting outside, both Ayrton and his paramedic were waiting in the lobby with their trolley and tethering.

"Let's fucking go," someone screamed as we charged into the cell... not really. The Police went first to try and press him up against the wall, they had shields and helmets, we forgot to bring ours. You don't think that clearly after a kebab and chips feast at 03:00.

Our job was to take over, using the four-man team tactics, I was number 4, head man and chief injector.

It worked pretty well, we shouted instructions at him while forcing him to the ground in various arm locks, we slipped around in urine desperate not to fall fully face first into it. My job was to push down on his wad of matted dreads and trip his legs, so we all fell down – in a controlled and graceful manner. He was incredibly strong and wildly screaming. I would have liked to scream also, like Braveheart going into battle. Yet, and unfortunately, there was an unwritten rule that only the patients could scream. If you did, you would forever have the piss ripped out of you – it would have been talk of the town for years.

Shame really.

So Rasta was in full technicolour surround sound fifth-gen Dolby®, and we were the monochrome slapstick silent movie, without accompanying piano. Not quite silent, we shouted at each other.

The big problem with giving a deep intramuscular injection to a wild stallion, is that it thrashes about in non-compliance. You then add to the mix the undignified and awkward removal of trousers and pants. This may involve reaching under the prone body to fumble around with a belt, zipper, or buttons, and then yanking down the clothing to reveal areas nobody wants to see, or smell, in the small hours of the morning. Dignity often went out of the window, although, to be fair, we did try. You have to mentally divide the full buttock into quarters and aim for the centre of the upper outer quarter, so as to avoid hitting the Sciatic nerve, or major blood vessels, go too high and you soon hit the hard bone of the Iliac Crest. Often your needle would snap and become lost in flesh, you then had to try and mark where it was, with a pen that you invariably didn't have, get another shot in successfully, and retrieve it later with tweezers from the tranquilised body. I was aware of patients walking around with three needles in them.

Also, Haloperidol Decanoate was oil-based - turns out to be Sesame - who knew? Get a Wok! It was a 'Depot' (meaning slow-release) substance, supposedly long-acting, and had to be administered by a 'Z-Tracking' procedure which took several minutes, it's aim being to spread and retain the oil base within the muscle, slowly releasing its active ingredients. Z-Tracking involved a stretching of the muscle between small and slow compressions of the plunger, stopping, releasing the muscle, going in a little deeper and repeating – two minutes was the recommended delivery time. The 'bright sparks' from above suddenly became hot on this once it was introduced, none of whom would have tried to tranquilize a thrashing wild horse over a two-minute period. The oily jabs were designed to be administered monthly but often we would find the recipient unwilling to receive it, and this ultimately would end up in the thrashing stallion scenario and you just get the oil everywhere except in the patient. You needed a thicker needle otherwise it was very hard to plunge the syringe, you sometimes needed two thumbs and gritted teeth. We needed the un-oily version - whack it in and be done.

When you're the jabber, the pressure's on. Everyone else has done their part, they are exhausted, barely able to maintain grips while maintaining awkward, painful, body positions (for both patient and staff) – and there may be added piss to contend with. If you fuck up by breaking the needle, or you can't push the plunger without getting sesame oil everywhere, you hear the groans of disappointment. You know it's going to come up in the debrief – and in the pub. If you balls-up the first attempt, the pressure just gets greater, then you near the awful experience of having to swap with someone else. (abject failure!) Swapping an armlock with another person is very complicated and likely to topple the cards – often someone gets hurt. You simply had to perform. Everyone watches your hands, hoping you are swift and successful, you know they are all looking, your hands start to shake, like an alcoholic in the morning, part nerves, part post-vigorous exercise, it happens with the finest.

On this occasion, I had an audience of at least eight. You would be advised to have your syringe ready primed with the cap on, knowing full well you would be using it within a few minutes. No idea why we didn't, so I found myself having to prime it with one knee across his buttocks and using his low back as a preparation table. So, you get your syringe, choose the correct needle, open that up by peeling the packaging then removing it, holding the plastic end, and sliding that end onto the opposite end of the plunger. The big risk was jabbing yourself or someone else. You then get your glass ampoule of five mg Haloperidol and snap it off at the scored line around the neck. This was tricky, if you held the top too tightly above the neck, the whole thing could crush between your fingers, it had to be a hard, fast, and confident snap. You needed to locate a little blue dot and have that face you as you snap away from it. It was a palaver. Paper towels between your snapping digits helped.

Then you had to load up the barrel, some people did this with the needle pointing down into the ampoule and drawing it up, others, like me, held the ampoule upside down, preying the meniscus and cohesion held the fluid inside, and sticking the needle up and into it. This reduced the bubbles you would create. And it looked cooler. You don't want to inject people with bubbles as that can cause an air embolism, and maybe kill the recipient, and one's career. So, you then had to repeatedly flick the upright syringe to encourage the bubbles to rise to the surface, so you can plunge them out. They are stubborn so you needed good flicking technique, it could take time.

Then you need to try and dispose of the glass ampoule before someone compresses it under their elbow... and jab the needle in without stabbing your fingers that are prising the skin taught. Whilst riding Rodeo.

Somehow, I did it without fucking up. Get In! (literally)

The writhing and screaming lasted another fifteen minutes, he was asleep by twenty. Most of us were full of cramp and desperate for a fag, or coffee.

Nope, no time for that, we had to strap him to the trolley bed, get him in the Ambulance (he was bloody heavy) and bomb back to base on blues and twos. To be honest we didn't use the twos initially. Blues = Flashing blue lights. Two's = Two tone siren which was the old 'Nee Nah, Nee Nah,' (for those who didn't know).

We had three in the back with the comatose body, two in the front including Ayrton Senna. Mission accomplished our errand complete. Detainee detained. Heading home in triumph, flags out.

Except he woke up.

Ten minutes into our homecoming, he stirred, moaned, and just woke up. We had about five miles to go. He started to flap about increasingly violently. Blood on his wrists from the plastic cuffs and the strapping started to come loose. It was just like watching Houdini hanging upside down in an aquarium. We were trying to keep him contained, not to be bitten or spat at, whilst doing 80 MPH in the leafy avenues of suburbia.

On came the 'Twos' and Senna dropped down the gears into maximum acceleration. We were flying but violently shaking from side to side, everything was coming loose. If anyone saw us pass by, we must have looked ridiculous, bouncing from side to side, like a lorry full of fighting wildebeest and hyenas.

There was a traffic speed control set-up near the hospital, two bollards, just wide enough to allow you through with inches to spare.

Go driver, go! Put your foot down man!

He did. We saw the bollards approaching rapidly, Ayrton's skill was not enough, we bounced sideways seconds before impact. It was a side impact (not too dissimilar to what actually killed the real Senna), but we then bounced into the other bollard with a heavy glance, our forward momentum got us through, but bodies were on the floor, I smashed my head on an Oxygen bottle. Rasta's trolley flipped diagonally, crushing someone's knee – but we got through and made it back.

The paramedic had radioed through, and messages got to the staff at the RSU and others on site in the hospital, we had around ten people waiting for us, one with a prepared syringe. As we fell out, they charged in.

Sometimes you just can't beat a four o'clock in the morning roll-up.

The Most Useless Present Ever

My time at this hospital was nearing its end. I heard that social services pay better than the NHS. I was getting tired of the shit. The inside of a locked unit containing nothing but grief and misery, bar the forced comradery we had to create to get through the shift. My panic attacks seemed to be getting worse, I couldn't cope in meetings in case I had to speak. Occasionally, I found myself in those situations where everyone had to introduce themselves to the group. As it worked around towards my turn, I would feel myself getting gripped with fear and a massive need to run away. Sometimes I did.

I had moved out of the nurses housing and into a shared house in Greenwich, South-East London.

At least I was with people who had normal jobs, albeit very boring sounding. But they were happy.

The most useless present I had seen before now was, as previously mentioned, the Filofax given to a severely handicapped individual with no obvious functioning parts, mentally or physically.

My leaving present even beat that!

I was a 'primary nurse' to a horrible individual who was your typical kiddie fiddler, didn't do anything more seemingly other than a quick fiddle wherever he could grasp the opportunity – like in supermarket queues. He was about four foot short, fat, and particularly ugly, with big thick glasses, a mouth breather with a fat tongue resting out on his bottom lip like a basking walrus. He thought he was 'all that.' Another deluded cretin. There was nothing to like about him. He thought we were mates simply because I would speak with him.

Nearing my departure, he would wink at me saying, "I've got such a lovely surprise for you Chris."

"Oh, Peter, I am overwhelmed with excitement, can't wait," I enthused.

My leaving day was nearing, nobody particularly cared. Some of my colleagues became good friends so I would continue to see them anyway. Otherwise, it didn't figure in the last few days. Except for Peter's increasing grin when he reminded me about his lovely surprise.

I knew he had been spending a lot of time in the woodwork room of the Occupational Therapy department and I was pretty sure he was creating a frame for a picture of himself. I knew that would be the kind of thing my colleagues (Barry, in particular) would have encouraged. It certainly would be the kind of thing a deluded cretin would do.

My last day came, and fairly uneventful it was apart from being confronted with a wild patient in the corridor who had just punched another patient, he was threatening further violence. We had assembled a quick three-man team to deck him and cart him off to seclusion. He was at one end of the corridor punching a window and we were at the other end.

"Look at you wankers, think you're hard don't you. Come on then," he beckoned a fight. He stood upright, stared at us, laughed, shook his head, and said, "You three make a right pair."

We collapsed in uncontrolled giggles.

Sixty seconds later he was dispatched into seclusion.

So that was my last shift. I was in the staff room, saying some goodbyes. Someone got a cake in, and they gave me a card.

Then Peter appeared at the door like the Cheshire Cat. Surprise!

He held out a large and heavy, square, and flat object wrapped in glossy colourful paper.

It was the size of a paving slab. Surely, he hadn't had his mug blown up that big?

As I unwrapped it, I could sense everyone looking on, most had no idea what it was. Barry was laughing.

I pulled out a large tile of plywood, rough at the edges, about two cm thick, the length of my forearm on all sides. As I ripped off the paper, I could see some extra chunks of wood stuck to one side. As I held it up in front of me, I started to make out that they were letters, badly jig-sawed. It took a while to work out which way was upright.

I made out an 'F' and then an 'I'. Ok, this way up then.

Holding it at full arm distance away, I began to work it out.

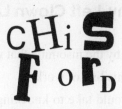

CHiS FORD

Ok, so a massive wooden plank with my name on it.

What does he expect me to do with this?

Who has the need for a badly made plaque of their own name?

Hold on a minute…, **CHIS!** WTF?!?, CHIS?!

I'm **CHRIS. CHRIS** with an '**R**'.

"**CHIS!** Ha ha ha ha ha!" – about three of my colleagues spotted it at the same time as they exploded in laughter.

Thirty years on, I am still called Chis by one of them.

There was a large rubbish skip, just outside the hospital gates, naturally I stopped next to it briefly on my way home.

Loony-Left Clown Land

I was still plagued by the insomnia that was caused by my very first shift in this line of work.

Sometimes I would take to knocking myself out with Whiskey in desperation at 04:00, and then get up and go to work for 07:30. This obviously wasn't sustainable, so I sought help with hypnotherapy. It was during a session that I had the realisation that violence, fighting and the threat of imminent injury was possibly something to avoid. Most people I know who work in that environment, don't do it for too long. Those who do, become addicts to something, look old before their time and are often miserable, angry individuals.

And divorced.

So, I figured Social Services, in the 'community,' would be less stress.

I was offered the job as deputy manager of a group home in central London, primarily for people with learning difficulties. I had no idea what kind of home, and with what level of 'difficulties,' I just got what they allocated. It was a couple of houses, knocked into one unit with around twelve residents. They were mainly profoundly 'disabled,' mentally and some physically. Some had sensory impairments while other characters were relatively able, the cheeky chap with Down's Syndrome, for example.

I turned up on my first morning looking and feeling like shit due to a long night of insomnia, but felt able to blag my way through, citing hay fever as my usual go-to excuse. The morning was at Social Services HQ dealing with HR issues, so I arrived at the house just after lunchtime.

It was their weekly staff meeting. Shit. All the staff were sat in a large circle in the lounge, around a dozen of them because we also had a smaller house on the same street. The meeting was timed to be between AM and PM shifts. I was invited in and John, the manager, decided to do the brief introduction circle, starting with Tony, on my left, going around further left, giving everyone their chance until it ended with me. Terrified. I could see them all looking at me. I could tell they were making their judgements. I had to say who I was, where I had come from and 'a little bit about myself,' as it was nearing my turn, I became overwhelmed in panic. At that moment I knew I had mental health issues. Imposter syndrome. Was I cracking up? Have I already cracked up? Am I going to end up as a patient? It did happen, in fact there was a unit at my previous hospital full of ex-psychiatric nurses and doctors.

'Come on man. Get a Fucking Grip.' I apologised for my hay fever, blew my nose to make me red in the face (a tactic I had used often before, migraine was the other, anything to explain my red face), and gave the briefest of introductions, but seemed to get away with it. They were all bloody looking at me though and I just wanted to run. Then John the big bald and very gay manager handed me a large red notebook. "Here you go Chrissy, can you read us all the minutes from last week?"

'You are fucking kidding!'

As soon as I saw the open page, and the three after, I knew this was going to be about ten minutes of utter hell.

"What... now?"

"Ooooh yes please Deary, I'm ready if you are." John minced his eyebrows and moustache in a 'take me now' fashion, an 'ooh matron' pout followed with a quick up-flip of the tongue and a swift ninety degree lateral head motion. His two hands up on stalks of fingers pressing on his crossed knee – you know the little routine. Nathan, his favourite squeeze piped up.

"Hands off you, he's mine." The room giggled. I was prey. Meat.

I pulled that kind of face you pull when you've realised you forgot to put your parachute on, just after exiting.

OK, head down and just read. Don't look at anyone, just read, get through it.

Most of it was like this.

'Martin said that Paul's feet seemed cold, Nigel agreed and said he noticed the same the other evening even though it was quite warm. All agreed that we should buy Paul some thicker socks or double up. Jane said that Keith had some he didn't use and suggested we lend them to him. All agreed that Keith would lend his thick socks to Paul.'

"Hold on just there Chris, lovey. Did you try this, Jane?"

"Yes, I gave them to Nigel."

"Any better Nige?"

"Yes, seems better now," said Nigel.

"Ok, carry on dear."

I was about five minutes in, just reading, face down. I just wanted to run away; I noticed the book I was holding was vibrating. Then, out of nowhere, a large drop of sweat plopped onto the page below me. I wiped it away and carried on. I could feel sweat really building up, running down my neck and my shirt sticking to my chest. I knew everyone could see me falling apart. I just kept wiping the sweat drops and sped up to the end. I was supposed to be the new deputy manager, the line manager for half of the staff present. I felt pathetic. Then everyone clapped and some cheered with sympathy.

"Sorry Chris; shouldn't have done that, but we do like to break the new ones in," John said, gesturing a wipe across his forehead with a,"Phew."

"Err, well thanks for the initiation," I said. I could see some staff were a little uncomfortable. "Hay fever's bad, seems to have kicked off a bit of a migraine."

And with that, I just sat and listened for twenty minutes

or so, feeling like a failure.

Somehow, and for no obvious reason, I regained my confidence and felt better as the day went on.

I kind of decided not to care, in fact I was a bit pissed off. I started to feel strength and a resolve to take charge of myself and had already hit a low point from the off – what was there for me to be afraid of now? I've been embarrassed and looked stupid but survived. Not caring what they thought suddenly made sense. It also took away the 'fear of failure' because, nothing actually happened. I didn't spontaneously combust! I just started to think in the great scheme of things that nothing on this level really mattered.

Social Services was weird, the people were weird. They were highly assertive and strongly (often wrongly) opinionated. They were all very 'right on,' all virtue signalling about stuff that seemed to really matter in the new loony left council paradigm. I heard about this as a 'thing' but didn't realise how full on it was. It was like working for a new religion, a doctrine, with thought police. Everyone seemed so aggressively gay. Everyone seemed to take offence. I was, bar one other, the only straight, white, relatively conservative, person there. I embraced this, but it was often pointed out to me as if, I shouldn't be.

I love people, I like all sorts of people and love to find their 'good' side, it's there somewhere in most. I like banter and piss-taking.

I love sarcasm and the ability to be cheeky, and for that to be received in the way it was intended. Not twisted.

I was never previously in a situation where I was surrounded by new rules of engagement that I didn't understand or knew about until I breached them. I mean I couldn't even imagine such a situation. Of course, it was entirely my fault for not knowing how I was supposed to think. Obviously, I came from a distant land from the dark ages, and in this world of Orwell's 1984 I needed re-programming.

The NHS psychiatric services have a slight military feel to it, you had to be hard and deal with banter. Nobody ever gave one shite if your 'feelings' were hurt. You would go out of your way to show you had no 'feelings.' Anyone complaining of 'hurt feelings' would very soon find themselves out of a job. If you can't hack it, you're in the wrong place.

Social Services, on the other hand was fully into 'Political Correctness' and the London Borough Council I worked for, were in the driving seat, devising new ways to be offended, new threats to one's feelings. It was as if a whole new mentality had been installed into local government. And to keep all of this in check, we had to fill quotas and tick boxes and compile reports, to prove the new way to think was being implemented. This was paramount and far more important than ensuring the service delivered quality care, to whatever it was serving.

I soon realised that my 'Mental Handicap' nursing qualification (RNMH) was not particularly important or valued. Not as much as being say, a black lesbian. Now, I can imagine lots of reasons to love a random black lesbian, but are they also able to write up a behaviour modification care plan for someone with Asperger's? No, especially if their previous management experience was in fucking Sainsbury's.

This is what was thrust upon us after John was sacked and imprisoned for stealing the resident's money – tens of thousands! Despite my bad first day, I had become a key stand-in manager and expected to step into the full-time role.

But, no, our regional manager simply had to fill the quota's, we needed more black lesbians.

Just to jump in here before y'all think I'm some kind of a white, right-wing racist, my girlfriend at the time was a beautiful black girl who later became my wife and mother of our two awesome kids, thirty plus years on we are still kicking!

The regional manager was a bloody disaster. I liked her in many ways, she was Welsh, said really shitty things in a jolly sing-along style. Once, when I was complaining about how little the new manager knew about anything relevant to the job, she reminded me that they needed my nursing skills so I could put a plaster on someone's painful bunion.

Her name was Daisy Brand, very 'right-on,' in her sixties, with purple hair and Doc Martin boots. She wished she was a lesbian, but I don't think her husband approved, so she just flirted, while at work.

She smoked for England, or should I say, Wales and spent ages in the manager's office with John, fugging the place up. None of us could go in there, even the smokers, it was as carcinogenic as Chernobyl but probably met health and safety standards due to a lack of trip hazards. They would smoke and talk about John's (anal) sex life with his husband Andy, and how Andy knows about Nathan but refuses to try a healthy threesome. I know this because John used to tell me.

He used to tell me way too much, but nothing about syphoning the resident's money into his and Andy's bank account. Until he got caught and sentenced, he called me all drunk and in tears just before his court case. Nobody knew and he could possibly have got away with it with a sudden disappearance or feigned death, but guilt got the better of him, he couldn't handle it and broke down in confession to Daisy over a fag.

God, I wish I were a (coughing) fly on the wall then. Imagine Daisy going from, "We're all gay mates here, loving it large," to, "oh shit, fuck, now I've got to do my job".

In tears, she called the police.

And John was Gohn.

Boxes Ticked

In came Candice Morrison, the shiny new manager, and everything fell apart. I remember, an excitable Daisy telling me they have found the new manager in the same breath as telling me my application was unsuccessful, her eyes lit up as she told me this lady had twelve years' experience running homes for people with learning difficulties, challenging behaviours, and some with varying degrees of mental health issues, how she had transformed these once underperforming units, with demotivated and disgruntled staff, and unhappy residents, how she had that magic touch as a trouble shooter, like the Hotel Inspector or Gordon Ramsey, revamping and re-energizing, making the phoenix rise from the flames…

Sorry, I got carried away in magic clown land there, rewind back to 'her eyes lit up,' should read thus; 'her eyes lit up as she told me she was black AND a lesbian!'

She did have great managerial experience though.

At Sainsbury's. The supermarket.

She seemed very much out of her depth on day one, seemed to drift off into a daydream when I tried to explain how things worked, and where things were kept, or recorded.

My initiation experience gave me a healthy bit of vengefulness, I think a little bit gives you the confidence to fight and to get the upper hand. Obviously, in general, vengefulness is self-destructive and the pursuit of unhappiness. Anger is an energy as the great John Lydon wrote, it is, and it can be channelled into a force for good if controlled. I was angry and vengeful, just enough to step outside of my social anxiety, which was good. I decided that I wasn't going to take any shit, and I'll just confront everything my inner radar perceived as wrong.

Porno Gangsta!

We had a lovely character, always smiling and cheerful (unless in one of his tantrums), a typical Down's – beautiful soul. We liked each other a lot and I would often take him out to watch football. Either the local topflight team, where he had a special membership + 1 (me), or to watch a local Sunday morning team with a player he knew (me). Sometimes perks do just come your way. I had one eye on the ball and one on Phillip, he would stand at the side of the pitch but would also wander off towards anybody with his hand and arm outstretched, offering his hand to shake in greetings. He would do that to everyone and often with one of my opponents preparing to take a throw-in. He would also decide to walk on the pitch to tell me that someone had the same colour jumper as him.

So, although I got to play every game, I also had to juggle my attention with Phil. It was nice to get paid to play football though. In fact, Sunday mornings were awesome, unless a particular South African lady was on shift. It would involve me totting up petty cash and other expenditure in the morning while the staff got the residents up, I would then give Phil a nudge to get out of his pit, make him his Jam sandwich, and off we would go for football. On our return the staff would have competed to make the best cooked breakfast. We had two kitchens to serve the two halves of the building. The breakfasts were always an epic multi-cultural event with the African Vs West Indian rivalry being the Champions League. Anything the whites 'knocked up' was always regarded as Vauxhall Conference – no spice.

I don't know how I got away with it because nobody knew I actually played. Phil tried to tell them sometimes, but he used to say a lot of wild, imaginary things – typical conspiracy theorist, often right but no one believed him!

If the South African lady was on shift, you would often find one half of the competition (her own) sabotaged, because she had gone into a wild rage – more on her later.

Phil's dad was a bit of an old wide boy, I liked him a lot. He clearly had underworld connections. He ran a porno video rental shop above a normal video rental shop. Well before the convenience of streaming such material. Phil's dad somehow had control of Phil's money, even though Phil was in his thirties. All residents had money from the government and generally, it would build up in an account because they really never used it. There were budgets allocated for all of their needs.

It was Christmas and Phil needed a new TV in his room. This was in the days when a fairly large screen TV was the size of a caravan. Phil's Dad, Ronnie, said he will get him a new one from the account as he gets good deals with a retailer. All agreed in the staff meeting that this was a good idea.

Christmas morning arrived, and so did Ronnie with a

massive box and two chunky blokes carrying it.

"£500," Ronnie said, "should have been six-fifty."

"Good job," said I.

Ronnie about turned quickly after a brief, "Merry Christmas Son."

I was excited for Phil. Actually, I was excited for me, I love opening presents, especially some cool tech. Brand new TV, at that price, was sure to have the latest kit. This was in the days when we had Ghetto Blasters, with 'V' shaped antennas and loads of knobs, like Treble, Bass, and Mid, or even a Graphic Equalizer! Graphic Equalizers always made things sound worse than the original mix, unless you convinced yourself otherwise based on it being a waste of time and you were fooled, which nobody wants to admit. So, you just had to create a 'wave' of sliders to impress your friends – who would always fiddle and change your settings, 'coz they know better about sonic science.

Anyway, the telly.

We took a kitchen knife to the box, sliding carefully along the middle length of sticky tape, and then flip, flip, under the lateral edges of the upper flaps – as you do. And 'Ping' it all unfurled like a flower.

At this point you expect to see a flat white expanse of polystyrene, tightly sat on top of the goods it was protecting, maybe with some clear soft plastic bagging and perhaps a pamphlet of sorts.

We found a jumper.

It was cuddling whatever it had below.

Woollen look but probably synthetic. Blue and white with diamond patterns, crew neck. I say white but more 'tobacco.'

Under the Jumper was the telly, sat on top of some toilet rolls.

We lifted the TV out and sure enough, it matched the picture of the Hitachi on the box. Under the TV, we found a remote, with no wrapping and a 'slightly thumbed' user manual. Clearly this TV had been used - and used for some time.

It worked ok, but there was no way it cost £500.

"Err, Ronnie, it's Chris, at Bolton Street," (we called the home by the name of its street).

"What is it?" his reply somewhat bellowing out of the receiver.

"Errr, have you got a receipt, per chance? For the telly?"

"Aint it working?" He said.

"Yeah, it works ok but…"

"That's ok then mate innit?" He interrupted, like he was forcing the end of the conversation.

"Errr, the thing is, Ronnie, I'm concerned it looks a bit, errr… second hand, kind o' thing."

"That's straight from the dealer that is, what you on abaaaaaT?" I could hear some spraying spittle at the aggressive 'T.' "I mean we tested it. What you saying?'"

Interesting to note how an East-End Cockney accent will usually drop the 'T's and 'H's.' So 'Hello' will usually be 'Ello,' and 'Fat' will be Fa (but with an abrupt end to the 'A' sound, done at the back of the throat, not using the tongue to make the 'T'.) The word 'Hat' would contain a pronunciation of neither the 'H' or the 'T.'

However, wind a Cockney up and they really go for it with the final 'T.' Sometimes adding a 'U' (as in the sound of the 'U' in 'UP'), after that 'T' – so, 'What You On AbaaaaaTU'

"Ummm, it's just that, well, Phil paid £500 quid for it and it doesn't seem like it's worth that kind of money - is it under warranty?" I replied.

"Listen mate, you'd better come down to the shop, let's sort it out here. And now," it was like he was challenging me to a duel. A bit threatening.

"What, on Christmas day?" Slightly hoping not.

"Yup."

"Thirty minutes."

As I was walking down the rough East-End road, I was mentally rehearsing my approach.

'Listen Ronnie, I think maybe there was a mistake, maybe they sent the wrong one?'

Or 'maybe you can just give it back, get your (Phill's) money back, and I'll just get him a new one in tomorrow's sales?'

I got there out of breath and then had to make my way up to the top floor once he had pressed the entry button.

As soon as I entered…

"'Ave you met Mick?"

Sat next to Ronnie was a very over-tanned, over hair-dyed gentleman, in an '80's black and orange track suit and dripping in heavy gold. The hair was that kind of black with a crimson hue. The eyebrows were also heavily darkened with the leftovers. There was a significant comb-over that appeared to involve some glue, and a flash of 'American' teeth that looked fit for a man sixty-five years younger than this. He was in his eighties. He had amazing skin, probably 'hide' a better term, old leather like a Chesterfield.

Massive gold rings on all fingers.

I knew instantly who he was.

Ronnie had backup. Backup with menace.

It's only bloody Mick Mc-bloody-Manus, out of the 70's. ITV wrestling superstar. Usually bouncing off the ropes to twat someone hard on the canvas in his blue leotard or sometimes just pants. He had fought everyone, Giant Haystacks, Big Daddy, Catweazle, Pat Roach, Davey Boy Smith, Brian Glover, Jackie Pallo… and the ultimate legend that was Kendo Nagasaki. I remember the great unmasking live on TV in 1977 – how exciting! 'World Of Sport' live from the Civic Hall, Wolverhampton. It was a ceremony, so the weird ring master announced – he, the ringmaster, was dressed in some weird panto garb, had dodgy eye makeup, and died grey hair. Ringmaster was also Kendo's manager, 'Gorgeous George.' Nagasaki was flanked by two monk-like 'acolytes of the inner circle of Nagasaki,' they had shaven bald front, top and sides but hair at the back, a hairstyle supposedly forbidden for anyone else! Apparently, Kendo had been in a secret retreat of meditation for months leading up to this ceremony, so 'o ringmaster one' said.

With that, Kendo got to his knees and planted a sword into the canvas – or whatever was covering the canvas to prevent sword damage. The two monkish chaps threw themselves, prostrate at his sides as salt was thrown in the air, then the ringmaster slowly removed the mask, up from the back of Nagasaki's head, revealing a tattoo of a pentagon with an 'all-seeing' eye in it on top of his skull, 'Hmmmm.' He then stood to reveal a good looking, but non-oriental chap – called Peter Thornley, with weird-coloured contact lenses. Sometime before, he was very nearly unmasked by Big Daddy, it was exciting stuff for me, who would have then been about twelve. The strain against strain to pull the mask off, I yelped in delight when we first saw the chin emerge, then the mouth in grimace, but it never actually came off, Kendo was too strong. We all knew it was a whole load of bollocks really, but it was better than playing with a hoop and a stick – ok maybe it wasn't that long ago.

Even more exciting, I've just read that Nagasaki shares the same birthday as me. Which is better sounding than the 'Michael Gambon' I previously cited on the odd occasion the subject would come up. I digress.

Mick fought them all.

And now Mick was here to fight me.

Why else was the legendary Mick McManus in a porn video shop on Christmas Day?

"'Ave we got a problem? – Christopher?"

"Look Ronnie, I think someone has ripped you off, maybe you didn't notice but there are scuff marks all over that telly and everyone's saying it's clearly not new. I don't want them thinking it's your fault mate, you know how people are, also the remote is a bit sticky, and there wasn't a receipt which we would need if there's any problem, maybe I need to bring it back to…"

"Are you saying I nicked it? I think he reckons it's 'knock-off,' Mick."

"No, no, no, no, no, no, I know you wouldn't do that mate, 'course, I just don't want people to think that, obviously, they gave you the wrong one, at your dealer, probably, mixed it up with one for repair?" For some reason I said the word 'repair' two octaves higher.

I mean I wasn't scared of being slam dunked on the office floor by an eighty-year-old, but was a bit concerned about any other 'boys' he may have in the back room. I imagined them sat round a poker table in a big cloud of smoke gagging to 'ave some of that'.

"Bring it back tomorrow, and I'll give you a Monkey," Ronnie said.

I sat for a while, trying to work out how to answer that. Did I hear correctly? What the fuck did he just say?

He then leaned in looking over his glasses, and repeated,

"Get it here tomorrow, and I'll give you a Monkey… Cash."

"Errr, have you gone all cockney rhyming, Ronnie? Coz, I don't know what that is."

"Monkey… five hundred spondoolies." (English Pounds)

Aha! Nice! So, very quickly I realised a Monkey wasn't a punch in the face and it was, in fact, him fully resolving the issue. Thank Gawd.

Mick gave me a prolonged hard squeeze handshake on the way out for some reason.

That Christmas night was one of my worst nights ever. I had a brief chat with my son, who I was missing, a lot. They were all together with extended family enjoying festivities. My shared house was empty, everyone had gone back from whence they came, it was big and silent. I finished around 10pm and decided to go home alone and drink myself to sleep. It's London, there was bound to be somewhere open. There wasn't, I drove all over, everything was shut. I gave up and went back to the loneliest place on earth knowing I was working again the next day at 07:00.

I felt so low, I could have parachuted out of a snake's arse.

PC World

Once John had been packed off to prison for embezzlement, and I had been ignored for the Managers job, due to not ticking the right boxes (there were only two), we had Candice from Sainsbury's (who ticked both) come in, to sort Bolton Street out.

It really needed sorting; the staff were like a herd of cats. Uncontrollable.

Daisy the regional manager popped in occasionally, but Candice didn't smoke and therefore there wasn't that camaraderie. Candice was dropped in at the deep end. And she drowned, bless her.

Within ten days, she went off sick, never to return. Guess who had to cover? A deputy manager deputised in the absence of a manager – they did not get paid a manager's salary whilst they were doing so.

One of my uses, by being trained to degree level in 'mental impairment,' was to know how to devise a behaviour modification care plan. We had many 'service users' with challenging behaviour. More often than not, they were very under stimulated, and this was very much due to the selfishness of a lot of the staff, who were also bone idle. Not all, but enough. The emphasis on cooking and watching TV 'with the residents' was self-serving. They would relish in the elaborate meals and simply couldn't miss Eastenders. If a service user made too much noise, they would be wheeled off somewhere else.

I would teach the staff how behaviour modification techniques worked if followed to plan. Simply speaking, we would ignore the bad behaviour - or intervene without any communication if the behaviour caused harm to others or themselves. Meanwhile 'good behaviour' would be rewarded.

I recently saw a dog psychologist on TV who was called in to try and help desperate owners of a dog who would just stare at its own reflection, in a catatonic state. They thought it had been possessed by the dog devil. It was quite disturbing to watch. The psychologist watched the owners and the dog in their lounge, the couple were sat on the couch watching TV. Sure enough, the dog went up to the glass doors of a cabinet and stared at its own reflection, close up, no movement. "Stop it Rufus. What are you doing? Stop doing that. Come here," the couple would say. "Rufus!"

After a short while, the psychologist knew exactly what was going on.

"OK, let's all walk out," he said. They had a camera set up. As soon as the owners walked out, the dog jumped up onto the couch.

"Right then sit back on the couch with Rufus, if he goes to the cabinet COMPLETELY IGNORE HIM."

Rufus sat there for thirty seconds before he jumped down in front of the cabinet and pressed his nose against his reflection.

The owners were desperate to say something, but the psychologist gave them a hard stare and gave the 'shhhh' sign.

After an excruciating five minutes the dog became a little confused, it withdrew from the reflection and sat looking back at its owners. A few minutes later it jumped up onto the couch.

"NOW! Give him attention."

"Well done. Gooooood boy."

They settled down quietly and watched TV for a few minutes. Rufus got up and went back to the cabinet. Stared at his reflection. Again, he was ignored. After just two minutes, he turned back and jumped on the couch.

"Goooooood boy. Well done!"

This process happened just one more time, thirty seconds in the reflection before he gave up.

Even a dog can learn quickly that their little trick to get attention didn't work anymore, he had been rumbled, the game was up.

The behaviour stopped just like that. The owners just needed to reward him with some attention when he was sat with them, doing nothing. The behaviour had been modified.

I spent a long time trying to deal with many challenging behaviours by writing up care plans that specified exactly how staff were to react. To the good behaviours as well as the bad.

The key is consistency. It takes much longer to break the cycle of expectation – behaviour – reward, than with Rufus but, eventually, you get there. The 'subject' needs to eventually realise their behaviour doesn't get the reward. For some poor souls their 'reward' was an absolute rollocking, it was still some attention and interaction.

In the early stages, when they don't get the usual instant bollocking, the behaviour increases in a more desperate attempt to get the attention. Eventually it would stop and then staff were instructed to reward the behaviour stopping with whatever reward worked. Some, who had the intellect would receive a star sticker that they could save up and exchange for a range of things, others may just get intense one to one attention, a puppet show, or a biscuit, whatever.

It nearly always worked. But not at Bolton Street. We would get so far, sometimes weeks into it, until selfishness and laziness cracked the resolve, and you would hear, "Stop it, stop it now, stop doing that, what's up with you? Why do you keep doing that? Stop it now," bellowing out of the lounge.

Brilliant, well done! Completely blown it, now they know just to push their food on the floor even more – or whatever the behaviour was.

I would try to tell Daisy how the staff were a fucking nightmare, and the residents challenging behaviours were increasing due to them not doing their job.

"Never mind, love, maybe you should have stuck to being a nurse. I want you to go on a 'cultural awareness' course next Thursday and can you complete this 'equal opportunities' form?"

I lost it and said, "Is this all you are ever concerned about? This place is a fucking nightmare and I get no support from you whatsoever – nobody has had any formal training, apart from all this PC shit."

I finished my shift immediately after that conversation. My girlfriend, now my wife thirty years later, was waiting outside so we could drive back to my flat. She got into the passenger seat and as we pulled out onto the road, she said, "Jeez are you OK? You look mad."

I was. "I fucking hate Daisy Brand," I said as I punched my own windscreen – it instantly smashed into an arial view of crazy paving. "Holy shit. Ooops".

Earlier in the day, I had hurt my back catching a falling resident. We had a tall chap called Tim with profound disabilities, who was completely blind, but he could walk, well, shuffle. He needed special one-to-one attention in case he decided to roam. That day I found him wandering just as he was keeling over backwards, it was a problem with his Cerebellum. His '1-1' had been called to attend a serious commotion in the kitchen where, apparently, somebody didn't season the rice properly. I caught him in md-fall and screwed my back and had been too busy to fill out an incident form.

My wife recalls that journey home. "I can remember it very clearly, I could see your face getting redder and redder, you were becoming more and more wound up, being confined in a car, that wasn't helping, you were swearing profusely and then, literally out of nowhere, you punched the windscreen, which shattered, smashed. I was in complete and utter shock, gobsmacked, I was worried about my own safety, got you to pull over and calmed you down." She then went on to say, "I found it quite a turn on to be honest, we had quite a physical night." (Sorry, kids!)

My back was obviously not too bad at first, but it sure came back to bite me later.

In fact, I took a couple of days off sick. Doing that jeopardised the whole unit because it was always understaffed due to 'staff sickness,' and we had to rely on agency staff who knew nothing about the residents or their care plans, so everything was just the bare minimum, if that.

Precious Metal

This South African lady was like a blob of Semtex – explosive, and as volatile as Uranium.

Precious Uranium Semtex, should have been her name, but it was Precious van der Merwe.

God help you, should you cross paths.

She would suddenly blow, regularly. I was informed by Daisy though, that she had heavy periods, and it was simply her cultural assertiveness (so she was female and black) and we would be wrong to question her 'attitude' or 'work ethic'.

Most of our unit's unacceptable sickness revolved around Precious, her 'heavy periods' (that we all had to 'picture' in our minds), meant one week off every month, but then she was also either pre-menstrual or post-menstrual, which caused so much bloody stress for everyone else that they would go off sick.

Her eruptions would shake the whole building and many a good staff member would crumble in front of her before handing in their notice. I would challenge her and then find myself being reported for racism. Daisy would have to discuss my attitude. Precious was precious. Daisy loved her, she was always so lovely and smiley in her presence. They would have virtue signalling competitions, who was the most politically correct, who was more 'Left and cool.'

This is how it would go with one poor guy (Jim), who always got it in the neck.

"Precious, is this rice dish done?" He may say in benign tones - meaning 'shall I start serving?'

"Are you saying I can't cook? Are you African Jim, Are you African? Are you a mother, Jim, are you a mother? How dare you say I can't cook. Did you hear that everyone, Jim think's it's ok to criticise my cooking, are you racist Jim?"

She would then go into a massive sulk and disappear, sometimes you would hear wails, leaving the rice to burn and set off the alarms. Jim had long gone.

I had to counsel Jim often, as his line manager, an impossible job, and then write out reports to send to Daisy, which were either ignored, or the follow-up questioning would be more about how Jim and I were perhaps insensitive to the 'bigger picture.'

Assertiveness - definition: Answering a simple polite question with another question, aggressively.

E.g., Jim: "Do you mind giving me a hand a sec, please, Precious?"

Precious: "Am I not entitled to a break, Jim? Am I not entitled? Do you think I am only here for you, Jim? Are you in charge here, Jim? What? Have you cancelled our breaks now Jim?"

It happened so many times that she once threatened Jim with some kind of a kitchen implement.

Eventually, Jim brought in his union representative and took out a grievance, which led to a tribunal that led to the eventual relocating of the now permanently sick Precious. Which meant she continued to not work, but to not work somewhere else. I had to give evidence at the tribunal and Daisy kept interrupting me to clarify and rectify the most minor, irrelevant points, such as exactly where the salt and pepper should be kept.

Fin

After the tribunal, I knew I was completely done with it all.

I was called into a meeting with Daisy to discuss my sickness – MY SICKNESS!

In the meeting it was pointed out that John's old flirt, Nathan, had objected to my overt heterosexuality, apparently the way I sat, with my legs apart, and folded arms, threatened him somewhat. FOR FUCK'S SAKE!

Daisy grilled me about both in the most patronising way possible, again degrading my nursing qualifications down to being able to put a plaster on a scratch.

I completely lost it; I really don't recall exactly what I said but it ended in 'FUCK YOU' and 'FUCK OFF', before slamming the office door behind me.

I walked across the corridor and headed into one of the bedrooms to calm down, I heard her also slam the office door and then the fire door at the top of the stairs. I heard her footsteps as she went down and out of the front door. She was smoking hard and obviously shaken. I watched her get into her car and drive off.

That was it, I knew my days in this mad job were over. But didn't know just how quickly and in what way.

I walked downstairs, turned the corner, and saw Tim, shuffling alone. It was then that a cruel form of divine intervention kicked in. Be careful what you wish for.

Before I knew it, Tim started to fall backwards. I instinctively leapt to his aid catching him, and his full body weight, as he accelerated toward the hard floor. My intervention worked out well for Tim, unfortunately, in one way, not so much for me. I let out one massive 'AAARRRGGGGHH' and, as Tim rose from the floor unscathed, I writhed around in agony before completely seizing up. Some staff came running to help.

"I've done my back in, shit. AAAARRRGGGH!" I howled, as one went to get ice and the other took Tim into the lounge, a third helped me to my feet and into the office where an accident form was filled out. Ever the professional!

I could feel like an electric shock in my lower back. "I need to go, get treatment, something, I need to go home now," I said pathetically.

One of the team offered to call an ambulance but I insisted I just needed to get to my car, and he helped me as I hobbled down the street like the Elephant Man, performed odd contortions to get in the car and slowly (but very surely) drove away. Strangely, my back pain momentarily subsided.

I felt like a mix between Thelma and Louise, an astronaut in a rocket blasting into space and a caged Condor breaking free and launching itself into the skies of the Andes.

I looked in the rear-view mirror and knew I wouldn't

be returning.

It felt Fucking Brilliant.

Massive smile on my face.

I just floored it.

I flew out of the Cuckoo's Nest.

PostScript

Despite actually being injured, I spent around six months constantly looking over my shoulder. If I felt there was any chance of me being watched by the 'department of malingering,' I would exaggerate my gait. The gait of someone with a bad back, which I had, I just didn't look like it. It started to interfere with my new-found, happy-go-lucky, do-as-I-please, life. In fact, I became somewhat paranoid. I was still receiving full pay, while sending in sicknotes stating the back pain, and some sciatica that I was experiencing. That period on full pay was coming to an end. Around one month after my accident, that coincidentally and not inconveniently happened immediately after telling my boss to Fuck Off, I received a formal demand to have an MRI scan on my lower spine to see if there really was 'a problem.' In their usual style they added two and two together, and came up with five suspecting I was conning them.

Around this time, I had noticed an article about Chiropractors, it seemed like quite a cool profession, certainly no stress that could compare to my last twelve years or so. I researched MRI scanning and what they could possibly see in my back, or not. I found it interesting so I applied for an interview, hoping my nursing 'degree' would be sufficient for acceptance.

I attended for my scan and waited. Obviously, my

worry was, they wouldn't see anything, while knowing that the malingerer tests a doctor carries out can easily be faked. 'Ooh yes that hurts,' and, 'No, my leg won't go much further up without horrible pain shooting down into my calf.' Luckily for me, in one sense, was that I never had much of a reflex when tested. The pain came and went but I looked OK.

I had re-mortgaged my flat when property values were hockey-sticking. I had cash to survive on but statutory sick pay would certainly help finance my Chiropractic training. Things would be difficult for me if I were sacked or forced back to work.

A few weeks later, the letter arrived from the Council (my employers). The MRI results were in. I had a disc prolapse at L5/S1 and it was compressing some nerve roots. Hooray! Not many others would celebrate such a result. Unless the alternative was an aggressive tumour, I guess.

I think the letter then said 'bla, bla' about working out ways in which they can help me, potentially a desk job, 'bla, bla, bla.' Suddenly, I could stop the paranoid limping, looking around to check for binoculars in the bushes, I had evidence! Yeeha! Unfortunately, I couldn't really sue for the accident as the MRI also revealed some arthritic changes that could easily cause the disc hernia. The Lord giveth then he taketh away!

My four-year (plus another – don't ask!) Chiropractic

course involved weekends and residentials, it was designed for those who also needed to work to sustain themselves (and pay for it).

To cut another long story short, to maintain my income, I did eventually go back to work for the council for a few years, they tried to get me to do some accounting bullshit desk job, forcing me to go for interview.

"So, why do you want this Job, Chris?"

"I don't, thanks."

I think it was the worlds shortest interview, they were slightly taken aback having previously sat in front of big-smiling, but desperate, "Yes, Yes, Yessers."

I was eventually given a part-time role at a very nice, generally happy, and relatively boring group home, while training to become a DC (Doctor of Chiropractic). Yes, there are a few stories, some really good ones, but nowhere near as big as what was to come in the future – that is for another day!

I understand that this book paints nearly all those described in it, in a bad light. There were lots of good people along the way, I just haven't concentrated on them here. Of course, all those I have written about had some good human qualities. So, it is important that I should acknowledge the brilliant characters and lovely souls I encountered during those years, both staff and inmates, residents, patients, and service users...

...Thank You!